Your Self-Healing Body:

Opening Avenues to Optimal Health

Daniel J. Dunphy, PA-C

www.biomedarts.com

DEDICATION

This book is dedicated to:

My family: my wife, Lynda, daughter, Ariana, and son, Ciancarlo, for helping make me a better human being.

My patients who are my greatest teachers.

Dr. Tom Laurence, whose kind yet persistent prodding has greatly improved the clarity and quality of my original text.

Praise for Daniel Dunphy and *Your Self-Healing Body*:

"We feel so blessed to have you in our lives! Our bodies most certainly have experienced healing because of your love, wisdom, treatment and guidance. You have led me to a path for optimal health. I have been successfully off all thyroid meds since February 2018 and my thyroid levels are now normal."

—Selena

"Very interesting philosophy based on experience, translated into scientific examples. Nice job, well done."

—Shimon Slavin, M.D.,
The Center for Innovative Cancer Immunotherapy
& Regenerative Medicine, Tel Aviv, Israel

"I just started reading this book and the more I read, the more my eyes start to well up with tears. It's just sooooo good!! What a brilliant and beautifully written book! It's a real work of art, full of digestible enlightening and empowering information. I am so excited that your wisdom is being shared in this way. You are truly making a positive difference in this world, and it's not just because of what you do—it's *how* you do it, with strength of character, with heart."

—Victoria

CONTENTS

A Deeper Understanding of Healthy

Whether you look with a powerful telescope into deep outer space or with a powerful microscope into deep inner space you will see patterns of reality that are present but often unnoticed, patterns in the everyday world around us. Galactic or atomic, planetary or cellular, when placed side by side these patterns all look very similar. They are fractal patterns. The parts and the whole are reflections of one another. When you observe nature closely these patterns are everywhere; the petals on a rose, the stems and twigs, branches and roots of trees, the swirls in the sand of beaches everywhere around Earth. This book is meant to demonstrate how these levels and patterns are working together to form life's self-healing nature.

Taking the time to listen long and well to your body leads to a deeper understanding of the patterns of imbalance that create symptoms of poor health. Through a deeper understanding of these patterns of imbalance you can uncover therapeutic handles that unlock your body's inherent healing powers. By removing blockages and supporting vitality, your self-healing body will open to do the real work.

CHAPTER 1

Your Self-Healing Body—Removing the Obstacles that Get in Its Way

Whenever patients ask me, "Can I ever get better?" I answer, "Of course you can, you're a self-healing organism." I mostly work with patients who have been through the ringer of medical treatments for chronic illnesses and have been washed through some of the gaping holes in theory versus reality, true understanding of multiple causative vectors versus the brand mark on their foreheads called diagnosis. It is to these people I address and dedicate these narratives. On the other hand, I have almost always found that I can reach people and touch the essence of their complaints by asking them, "What are your priorities? What do you want to achieve?" Connecting here then listening well and long opens the door to expressions of injury and suffering, past and present, physical and emotional. Listening to story opens you to deeper understanding with the opportunity to begin feeling better within a few weeks to months. I never drag anyone into something they're not ready for. I do not expect them to understand what I tell them in a single 2-hour session. I encourage them to record our conversation, ask questions, and send emails or text follow-up questions. I want them to grope, to be challenged, to grow if they are willing to do so. I grow with them. If I sense that they are not ready I will tell them that I don't want to waste their time or money. Neither do I want to waste my own with the impossible task of reaching everyone.

Often, to achieve this healing response, you must remove a blockage or a number of blockages to allow your body to heal. This could be anything from a rotten tooth, a scar, a gallstone or kidney stone, an infection, a clogged artery, releasing old trauma, or addressing a rotten emotional life. Removing the blockages releases the healing response. When you experience even a glimmer of positive turnaround, this experience serves as a handle you can grasp to pull yourself out of an impasse. Even though little has changed you still have the overwhelming feeling that you're going to get better. This is the therapeutic handle, the fractal that releases healing. It is flipping a downward, "down the drain" spiral into an upward, "going to get better" spiral.

A fractal is a part that mirrors the whole. A hologram is a 3-D photograph made up of light fractals known as photons. An example of a hologram is the little bird image on a credit card. Fractal geometry is the mathematical expression of the holography inherent throughout Nature. Fractals are parts of a greater reality whose form reflects and is reflected by the whole. If you were to look at a holographic plate and you illuminated that plate with a diffused laser light, you'd see an image like the ones on your credit card. You'd see dimensionality. You could look around the image to see the sides of the 3D image. If you took that same holographic plate and directed a narrow beam of laser light through just a point on the plate what would you see? A part of the image? No. You would see the entire image but with less detail, less density of photons. So photons, by their nature, when coherent, as with laser light, (meaning in-synch wavelengths of light), collect and reflect as much information in an instant as reality can dish out. The narrow laser beam diffuses holographically in space-time. Less photons create less detail. When the laser is diffused over the entire plate all the photons fluoresce. Here as everywhere in nature the part contains the whole and the whole the part.

A key to understanding this phenomenon lies in understanding that the Universe is fractal (the same patterns reoccur at different quantum scales) and holographic (the whole is contained in the part and the part in the whole, everywhere and within everything). Finally, the Universe is synergetic (the whole is greater than the sum of the parts). Your self-healing body is a reflection of our fractal, holographic Universe. (To further understand these concepts, visit **cosmometry.net**)

As with many things, the way we look at reality opens or closes windows of perception. We observe fractals not just on credit cards or in holographic photography but throughout Nature's self-organizing creation, from pine branches to pine trees to pine needles to the micro-organisms and insect life which are symbiotic with the pine tree.

Holography and fractal geometry and mimicry are everywhere in daily life, if we open our eyes to the wonder of their presence. See if you can tell which of these photos is a Hubble deep space photo and which is human blood:

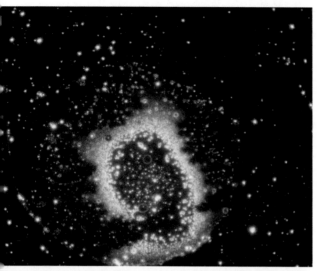

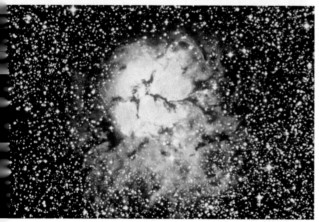

As you can see, whether you are in deep space on a galactic scale of reality or whether you're in deep inner body space, light year or micron quantum reality, the organization of fractals into structures is emerging at all levels, in our own quantum level of meters and kilometers as well as on our planet, solar system, galaxies and universe. Just as every quantum level emerges and builds upon the quantum below, so healing in our body reflects the same profound structure and holography. Holography exists in the fractal expression of cells in your body that hold your particular hologram and act together to keep you alive and healing.

When my patients see the living image of their blood under a dark field microscope, I remind them that, "All those millions of individual cells you are seeing are all you. They have your imprint; they act in unison to maintain your equilibrium and your life. When they ail, you ail. When your consciousness is distressed, they become stressed, and when you act in healing ways, they heal."

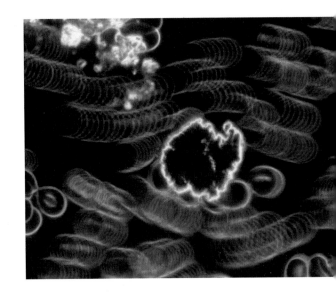

It's true, our bodies are self healing, from the inside out and from the cellular level up to organ and structure levels and, of course, in mental, emotional and spiritual levels. There is a fractal and holographic nature to healing which underlies your own life experiences of getting better, returning to normal, getting your energy back. For example, if you cut your finger and a week later it has healed and then you start using your hand again and you're no longer in pain, or if you make a positive change in your life and you start feeling positive about going on, you are experiencing the self-healing nature of your body. These little changes and healings reaffirm and motivate you in your life every day. The same is true for every other person on the Planet. In fact, the human condition is to push on even though we all know someday our body will wear out. Many would acknowledge that this defines courage and heroism. Those with illness who push on against all odds are true examples of this courage. The experience of everyday healing, the frequently unnoticed reality of nature's self-organizing ability is the spark that keeps the human spirit alive, that ignites your will to push on in the face of adversity. Seen from this perspective you can observe how your body reflects a greater cosmic reality. Your body is a reflection of this universe you have emerged from and into which you will be recycled when you go through the reverse birthing process humans call "dying."

Later this book will present you with three actual cases of the body's self-healing nature and the wonder of releasing that energy when it is blocked. Several states of imbalance, discomfort and what is called disease will be described. These case studies will demonstrate how similar conditions of imbalance can lead to many different expressions labeled disease. In spite of the labels humans use to understand and describe disease states, all states of health and dis-health just like all biological systems are constantly changing and evolving towards self-organization or chaos, stasis or vitality, life or death. You can alter your energy states by the life choices you make. You can choose to change for worse or for better. Many diseases that medicine calls chronic degenerative disease are in fact reversible states of chronic metabolic imbalance. If you see your life decisions including diet, emotions and life styles as either contributing to physical problems or helping solve physical problems then you can help resolve rather than create problems. How you think about things determines how you affect reality including your health. When you open your eyes to changing your state of health, you can begin to change your life. You begin to change the smaller picture from which your days emerge into a bigger reality of sharing life with all living beings on a small planet revolving around a small star on the edge of a swirling galaxy in an ever-expanding cosmos.

Look again at the photos of Hubble deep space photography and photos of living human blood. You will see many similarities, self-organization and entropy (loss of energy and structure) that reflect levels of energy within each system. We are located between these systems, macro and micro. Your self-healing body is a part as well as a reflection of the link between stars and cells, galaxies and atoms, the cosmos and your cure.

 Take Home Points

- Often, to allow your body to heal, you must remove a blockage or a number of blockages.

- If you see your life decisions including diet, emotions and life styles as either contributing to physical problems or helping solve physical problems, you can then help resolve rather than create your health concerns.

CHAPTER 2

Does Your Body Have Enough Energy To Heal?

Yet, there is more. Your body also requires nourishment to gather the energy to mount a healing response. So healing requires not just attention to your anatomy and your emotions, but also to your level of energy, commonly called vitality. When you are born your vitality and life potential are often at their pinnacle. As time goes on you will begin taking on life's stresses, the emotional-situational stresses, the traumas, chronic injuries, pain, infections and allergies, and finally the glycemic/insulin stresses or blood sugar challenges. Over time inflammations can turn into chronic degenerative conditions. For instance, frequent respiratory infections can evolve into chronic bron- chitis or asthma and in this process your body's energetic state decreases. The process of energy loss can be located within an organ, within a system, but the loss always interacts with the entire body. In order for your body to mount a successful healing response you have to have adequate resources to make that leap. Like a salmon swimming upstream to spawn, your body's energy systems must be adequate to make the jump to a better state of health. Here is an illustration of the process—a double spiral of healing energetics:

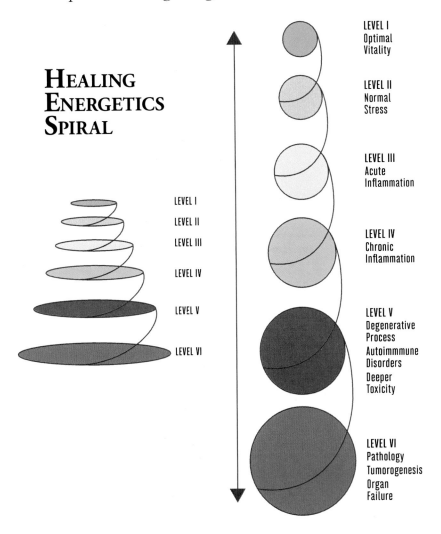

HEALING ENERGETICS SPIRAL

LEVEL I
LEVEL II
LEVEL III
LEVEL IV
LEVEL V
LEVEL VI

LEVEL I
Optimal
Vitality

LEVEL II
Normal
Stress

LEVEL III
Acute
Inflammation

LEVEL IV
Chronic
Inflammation

LEVEL V
Degenerative
Process
Autoimmmune
Disorders
Deeper
Toxicity

LEVEL VI
Pathology
Tumorogenesis
Organ
Failure

Where does this energy to heal come from? If you say energy comes from food we eat, the water we drink, the air we breathe you'd be partially correct. The quality of the food and water we consume and also how well our digestive track transforms that food into usable forms of nutrients are surely both critical to maintain a good energy state. There is more of course.

Think about how you start your car. You place the key in the ignition and turn the starter motor, this sparks ignition and the voltage regulator manages how much energy is used by the system, how much charge is drawn from the battery and how much energy is generated to recharge the system. Your body's starter motors are the adrenal glands located over your kidneys, the voltage regulator is the thyroid gland located midline in your neck, and your body's generator battery for energy generation and distribution occurs mostly in the liver. This energy generator and distributor are a biological cycle of electron capture and distribution called methylation. In chemistry, methylation concerns methyl groups, [CH3-], a carbon atom bound to 3 hydrogen atoms. As in all biochemical unions, form creates function. The methyl group [CH3-] is an electron-charged, biochemical micro battery molecule. These charged molecules known as SAMe distribute electron energy into every cell in your body. Once absorbed from protein you eat, the liver uses methyl groups from the amino acid methionine to make SAMe. SAMe molecules prime the mitochondria energy factories within every cell of your body with electron energy. SAMe enables production of the energy molecule ATP and brain neurotransmitter production that affects your mood and cognitive ability. SAMe allows your cells to eliminate toxic free radicals and regulate genetic expression. Look at the methylation/generator chart to see the entire cycle.

When your body tries to address chronic degenerative illness, all three of these systems—adrenals, thyroid and methylation—need to be functioning well. If you crank the starter motor and the battery is weak or dead, your engine will not only fail to

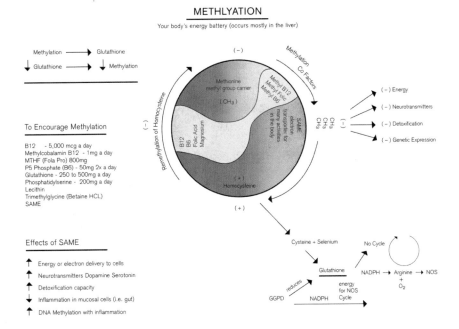

METHLYATION

Your body's energy battery (occurs mostly in the liver)

Methylation ⟶ Glutathione

↓ Glutathione ⟶ ↓ Methylation

To Encourage Methylation

B12 - 5,000 mcg a day
Methylcobalamin B12 - 1mg a day
MTHF (Fola Pro) 800mg
P5 Phosphate (B6) - 50mg 2x a day
Glutathione - 250 to 500mg a day
Phosphatidylserine - 200mg a day
Lecithin
Trimethylglycine (Betaine HCL)
SAME

Effects of SAME

↑ Energy or electron delivery to cells

↑ Neurotransmitters Dopamine Serotonin

↑ Detoxification capacity

↓ Inflammation in mucosal cells (i.e. gut)

↑ DNA Methylation with inflammation

turn over, you'll eventually fry the starter motor. How often have you heard the expression, "I'm fried." Or "I'm burnt out."

When you use a crutch such as sugar or caffeine to support your starter motor adrenal glands you're taxing all the systems and organs in your body. The thyroid and methylation can weaken and so your energy capacity is diminished, your capacity to detoxify is diminished and your overall sense of well-being and frame of mind are weakened as well as your ability to heal.

Take a look at what I call the "Holosystemic Mandala." It illustrates what I have just stated. Cortisol, which is your body's universal response to any form of stress, arises from the three major categories of stress:

1.) Emotional/ situational stress.

2.) Inflammatory stress: pain, trauma, allergic reactions, insomnia and infection.

3.) Dysglycemic stress—glucose/insulin imbalances

Take Home Points

- When your body tries to address chronic degenerative illness, all three systems—adrenals, thyroid and methylation—need to be functioning well.

- Avoid using sugar or caffeine as a crutch to support your starter motor adrenal glands, otherwise you're taxing all the systems and organs in your body. The thyroid and methylation can weaken and so your energy capacity is diminished, your capacity to detoxify is diminished and your overall sense of well-being and frame of mind are weakened as well as your ability to heal.

- Balancing your cortisol levels is critical if you want to have optimal health. Chronic cortisol overloads can have a negative impact on your body's self-healing pathways.

Look at the Mandala and notice how cortisol is at the center because from the beginning life is work and stressful. Cortisol is your survival hormone, and cortisol interacts with all your body's systems. Imbalance and symptoms of distress show up differently in each of us depending upon multiple factors including genetics, your own personal constitutional strengths and weaknesses, what infections, traumas and injuries you have suffered as well as how you live and where, not to mention your attitude towards these life experiences. Cortisol interacts with and aids your body's ability to adapt to stresses—going fast to catch food or going faster to keep from becoming food. This is why cortisol is positioned in the center of the Mandala. Chronic cortisol overload creates chronic negative feedback loops that can interfere with and affect every system in your body. Chronic cortisol overloads can have a negative impact on your body's self-healing pathways, but more on this later. For the moment I just want you to see the Mandala.

THE HOLOSYSTEMIC MANDALA
An Owner's Guide For The Human Body

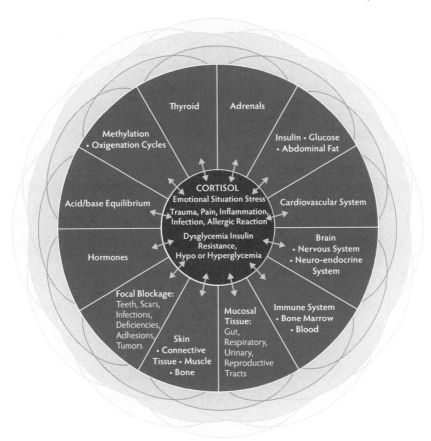

Your Self-Healing Body in Action

Case Study #1:
Reducing the Uncomfortable Side Effects of Estrogen-Blocking Drugs in a Breast Cancer Patient

A 51-year-old patient whom I will call Barbara first visited my office in 1997. I have been helping care for her for the last 18 years. She came to me a few years after she had been diagnosed with a type of breast cancer known as DCIS (ductal carcinoma in situ). About 40 percent of these localized cancers mutate into a more aggressive IDC (invasive ductal carcinoma of the breast). Adenocarcinoma is a type of cancer that occurs in mucosal tissue, as found in the milk ducts of the breast, the colon, pancreas, gallbladder, lungs, kidneys and reproductive organs. Adenocarcinoma is inherently inflammatory, inherently mutagenic, and inherently grows blood vessels to allow both growth and spread. Adenocarcinoma cells outpace normal cell growth and can grow dramatically for growth's sake. It is an oncogenetic parasite or parallel organism whose genetic software takes over normal cell functions and then goes on a joyride, crashing normal cellular function and normal body ecosystems. It also has survival and proliferation strategies that drive metastasis into the blood stream and lymph system. These features often make adenocarcinoma lethal. Women do not succumb to lumps in the breast but rather to the lethal seeding of cancer cells to vital organs like lung, brain, liver and bone. Luckily, in Barbara's case, the cancer was diagnosed before it had reached that point.

Before her diagnosis, Barbara had regular mammograms and she had no family history of cancer. Ultimately, the mammograms failed to detect the tumor. Barbara felt a lump at 4 or 5 o'clock in the lower outer quadrant of her left breast, near her armpit, during a self-breast exam. Barbara reported the lump to her doctor, who ordered an MRI and an ultrasound which confirmed the presence of a mass on her breast. A biopsy revealed Barbara had DCIS. Six months prior to her first appointment with me she had undergone a lumpectomy in her left breast but had refused chemotherapy and radiation.

A Quantum Approach to Cancer Treatment

The majority of people including the medical profession think of cancer as a lump, or a lesion, a discreet object that can be pinched or poked, biopsied then fried or poisoned to be rid of. The reality is that cancers are a failure of the immune system as well as the entire ecosystem of the body to identify and eradicate what is essentially a molecular or rouge DNA parasite. Cancers are generated by molecular, DNA mutations and these mutations or alterations have multiple causes. In addition, the tumor is an expression of the cancer, not the cancer itself. Once a tumor has become large enough

THE IMPORTANCE OF SELF BREAST EXAMS

Performing a self-breast exam once a month is critical to detecting malignancies. For all the technologies we have, there is often nothing more sensitive than your own sensation of what's normal and what's abnormal. When you do a regular self-breast exam you get to know what your breasts normally feel like. It is much easier to detect an abnormality if you are aware of what feels normal through regular exams. Breast exams should be done when you're not menstruating. Ask your medical practitioner to show you how to perform a self-breast exam and then practice it monthly.

to show up on a scan it already has 400 to 700 million cells. What's more, a person who has had a metastasizing type tumor will continue to have circulating tumor cells the rest of their life. This is true whether or not another lump ever shows up again. Many cancers are not benign. Many can potentially kill their host in an aggressive survival struggle whether treated or untreated. When I see patients who are undergoing treatment for cancer, I try to bring into focus three big goals for a sustainable outcome:

1. Containing future systemic cancer expression in long range, life-preserving ways and educating the patient and their family about the nature of what they are dealing with in order to make more informed and rational decisions

2. Encouraging detoxification and elimination of cancer-causing, immune-suppressing substances and conditions

3. Tonification or enhancing a person's vitality in order to help my patient mount an adequate healing response.

Conventional oncology follows protocols of pharmaceutical approaches to cancer treatment targeted at shrinking observable tumors. The normal procedure is to feel or find a lump, biopsy the lump, look under a microscope and identify the morphology or cellular characteristics then look at approved pharmaceutical interventions many of which have short-term success and long-term failure. If it looks a certain way under a microscope, a specific diagnosis is made based on location and morphology. This cellular diagnosis then generates a protocol for treatment relying upon organ-based categories of understanding cancer.

However, the problem with this approach is that in order to manage cancer with any long-term level of success, there need to be different quantum levels of analysis. The first quantum level is the macro level, the level where a lump is detected. The resolution limit of a PET/CT scan is 4mm. The average size for a mass to show up on the most advanced scan is about 7mm. A 1cm mass contains about 10 billion cells, a 1mm mass contains about 100 million cells. So, a 7mm mass must contain about 700 million cells to show up on a scan. That's a lot of cells. The cancer has taken over cells of the breast then churned out clones that have gone for a joy ride of fast growth and inflammation, and it has gone way beyond the single cell mutation from which it originated.

Another quantum level is the microscopic level. This is at the level of microns rather than millimeters. It's a thousand times smaller. At this microscopic cellular level, single cells and the morphology of the cells are visible. Abnormal morphologies are reflected in cancer for many reasons. They tend to be pleomorphic, that is they tend to have many irregular shapes. Tumor cells are experimental clones vying with one another as well as surrounding normal healthy tissue. They're usually not as symmetrical as normal cells are and they stain differently than normal cells under the microscope. In this case of adenocarcinoma of the breast, the tumors are usually lobulated, in other words, there are multiple fingers coming out of the mass. That type of morphology or outward appearance at this cellular micron level is suspicious for cancer.

The third quantum level of analysis is at the molecular level. This is done on a nanoscale by analyzing the intracellular molecular DNA, where the cancer originates. Cancer originates as a molecular, oncogenetic disease. It's a molecular quantum parasitic disease that parallels the body's own metabolism, inhabits it and derives its vitality from it. All kinds of different factors cause mutations in DNA including radiation exposure, heavy metals, pesticides, trauma, our own constitutional ability to fight off cancer and our ability or inability to detoxify. These factors are all tributaries that lead into the diagnostic river called cancer.

Breast cancer is one of the few cancers where the tumor is regularly analyzed both at the micron level using a biopsy, and also on a molecular level. Yet, this is done in an incomplete manner. The reason why breast cancer tumors are studied on the molecular level is that there are therapies that can target specific genetic level growth factors. Genetic pathology tests are used to determine whether the breast cancer is estrogen positive, progesterone positive, or HER2/neu positive. These are oncogenetic markers for which there are targeted therapies. In Barbara's case, her tumor was strongly estrogen positive. What this means is that Barbara's cancer genetics—the cancer software—included a receptor on the cancer cell for estrogen. Therefore, estrogen is a growth factor for Barbara's cancer. This is the most common type of receptor on breast cancer cells.

The reason why breast tumors are studied at this molecular level is because the molecular markers that tell the oncologist whether a tumor is estrogen positive, progesterone positive or HER2/neu positive can determine which drug therapies should be used to put ankle weights on the ability of the cancer to grow. For estrogen-receptor positive tumors, estrogen-blocking drugs, usually tamoxifen or aromatase inhibitors such as anastrasole (Arimidex®) are used. Herceptin®, a monoclonal antibody treatment, is used to shut down the HER2/neu receptor site on the cancer cell.

The problem with these treatments, however, is that nature doesn't use single genes. Cancer is inherently mutational; there can be many more chromosomes in cancer cells versus 46 in normal human cells. Being mutational, cancer can go down many different pathways of mutation. Therefore, estrogen-blocking therapies can not only

WHAT IS HER2/ NEU-POSITIVE BREAST CANCER?

When a breast cancer is HER2/neu positive it means that it tested positive for a protein called human epidermal growth factor receptor 2 (HER2). This protein is involved in cancer cell growth.

cause great discomfort in patients using them but the cancer can also mutate and develop resistance. That's what cancers do best. In order to survive, cancer uses multiple pathways through trial and error. This is why a tumor is not the cancer but a downstream manifestation of something that started at the nanoscale of DNA mutation. The tumor is a downstream expression of cancer's molecular mutation process. The software of the cancer occurs at the molecular nanoscale and is expressed at the cellular level in what's called a tumor.

A Flawed Cookbook Approach

The norm in oncology is to first perceive a mass, take a biopsy, look at it through a microscope, make a diagnosis based on morphology then go to a cookbook and proclaim the cancer comes from a certain place in a certain organ, then follow established treatment protocols. This clinical process often bypasses the molecular level, the quantum level from where the cancer has originated. These days some molecular testing has become normal yet not expanded enough to allow for more individualized care. So, it's not an individualized treatment. It's a cookbook approach and it's often a recipe for disaster because when treatments target only one or two genetic characteristics, this can and often does train the cancer software to adapt and mutate to survive. In a Darwinian sense we are often training a cancer *mutanome* (the complete mutational genetic code) to become more resistant, more aggressive and more likely to spread over time. This is especially true if the particular cancer oncogenes of an individual don't match the statistical norm of cancer treatment protocols. Unfortunately for many patients this is often the case. It's a morphological analysis and a statistical treatment. There is no other branch of medicine where that would be acceptable. In any other branch of medicine, you culture and test before you treat and repeat the process more thoroughly if treatment has not been successful.

Here's an analogy for the process used to diagnose and treat cancer and at which quantum scale it's being analyzed. I see a ship 30 miles off the coast on a clear day, and I look in my logbook, which indicates that because it's this day at this time of year there's a 65 percent chance that boat is from China carrying rice. Consequently, I'm going to treat that boat as if it's a Chinese boat with rice on it. But if I take out a pair of binoculars and look at that ship and it's an Australian ship carrying kangaroos I'm going to treat it differently.

Similarly, in cancer diagnosis and treatment that ship would be the cancerous mass. The mass is examined at the cellular morphological scale and then a statistical analysis is done based on the average person with that type of mass over time, and a statistical treatment—a cookbook treatment—is prescribed. But if you examine the ship more closely with a pair of binoculars—in this case a molecular scale analysis—it allows examination of the cancer software, of the genetic mutations the cancer is using to survive at a particular person's expense. By examining the genetic software of the cancer an individualized treatment approach becomes possible. The science and technology of making more sophisticated and complete oncogene analysis is already here. Unfortunately, clinical application of these technologies is years behind the science.

I'm not talking about observing just one or two of the mutations that have occurred that are part of the cancer software but the entire mutanome, meaning the entire cloud or complex of mutations that are in the back pocket of this cancer. The mutanome is essentially a software program that allows the cancer to manipulate cells away from functional normal growth, turning the cell into a power factory for growing with no differentiation and no purpose other than survival— growing blood vessels, causing inflammation then feeding off inflammation, shutting down immune function, and disguising itself—a stealth weapon allowing cancer to become the wound that doesn't heal. But if the wound that doesn't heal doesn't happen to fall into that 65 percent of ships that are coming from China at this time of year carrying rice, if you don't fall within the sweet spot of that rather narrow statistical bell curve, then you're out of luck because the treatment you're going to be given will not be effective. In fact, it may actually train the cancer to get worse.

One reason for this is the presence of cancer stem cells, also known as EMT cells (endothelial to mesenchymal transition cells). These cells have characteristics of normal stem cells but will always remain cancer seeds circulating in blood and lymph and awaiting a call response from the microenvironment of an organ. Once implanted the EMT cancer stem cells transition back to an endothelial form and grow into more tumors. These cells are not as vulnerable to chemotherapy as clonal tumor cells. They represent the spreading potential of cancers and can and do adapt to chemical as well as targeted therapeutic strategies. The patient will then slide down a slippery slope with a more aggressive, well-trained, and adaptive cancer than they had originally. That's the Achilles heel of oncology. We need to understand this fact to succeed in containing cancer growth over time. The science of cancer biologies is growing rapidly and intricately and promises many new biological approaches.

How I Worked with Barbara

I'm interested in helping patients contain the cancer over time by supporting their immune systems, by gentle and persistent detoxification therapies as well as supporting their overall vitality, helping them to survive medical interventions and importantly have a better quality of life and outcome. The science of autologous vaccines which use an entire cancer genome combined with activated natural killer cells harvested from the patient can train the immune system to target and unmask some cancers. Successful biological treatments and management of cancers are the future and they have arrived.

With cancer patients I mainly want to listen to their story, review their scans, blood tests and treatments but also discuss the nature of cancer biology, encouraging them to make therapeutic decisions out of information rather than out of fear. I have had many conversations with Barbara of this nature over the years. I also discuss three goals with her and with other patients:

1) *Containing cancer expression*: Containing cancer over time in the most sustainable and successful ways. This includes resourcing potential trials that match a patient's oncogenetic profiles.

2) *Detoxification*: Gradual and well-timed detoxification and elimination strategies that address factors that may have and continue to contribute to cancer. This includes assessing toxic exposures such as heavy metals and pesticides and understanding the ability of the person's methylation capacity as well as a person's constitutional ability to detoxify, inherited strengths and weaknesses. Emotional support, somato-emotional release and laughter are all important as well. In short, we aim to identify and eliminate stress factors, which get in the way of the body's innate healing capacity. That includes toxic relationships, toxic work environments, bowel ecosystem health, anything stress related. And it's important to go beyond detoxification, which is shaking the dead leaves off the tree. Equally important is encouraging elimination. This is like raking up the leaves and composting them, encouraging the body to cleanse itself naturally. Saunas, bathing, juicing, bowel and liver cleanses and drainage remedies are often employed. In very real ways our bodies are composting organisms, in the bowels as well as other organs and tissues, in

the blood stream, and in inherited, cellular immune function. Our bodies compost toxins and recycle them and when our bodies are overwhelmed by toxic stresses the result is imbalances that can lead to disease states. Compost or be composted!

3) *Tonification*: tonify or strengthen a person's vitality so that they can mount an adequate healing response no matter which therapies are selected. Aim to strengthen the organs of elimination and the immune system. That includes supporting the liver, the intestines, the lungs, the lymphatic system, the kidneys, and the adaptive or cancer-fighting aspect of our immune system.

Addressing the emotional aspects of toxicity is critical as well. Cancer can appear or increase dramatically in people who have lost a loved one or a pet or had some large emotional trauma. Within a year, cancer shows up statistically much more commonly after the loss of a loved one. Do emotions cause cancer? No, not any more than a tributary by itself causes a river, but it's often a trigger mechanism. Emotions and emotional trauma increase cortisol, a survival hormone that interacts in a negative way with every system in the body including chronic inflammation, methylation, immune function, sleep, etc. So often emotional factors are the trigger that pulls a loaded gun.

I kept each of these goals in mind when Barbara came to me with her breast cancer diagnosis. However, after lumpectomy, the main tool to contain more cancer expression—the estrogen-blocking drug tamoxifen—gave Barbara such severe side effects that her oncologist finally stopped estrogen-blocking therapy. If we were to achieve the first goal of containing the cancer over time, we would need to reduce those side effects so that Barbara could continue to take the tamoxifen. Because tamoxifen has the potential to cause cervical cancer, it was also important to try to reduce that risk. Tamoxifen blocks the growth receptor sites for estrogen on the cancer cells by occupying those receptor sites that estrogen attaches to. For this reason, women who have estrogen-positive breast cancer are prescribed the drug for five or more years after the tumor is removed. Because tamoxifen is an estrogen blocker it often throws a woman into menopause. This is what happened to Barbara a week after she had been taking the recommended dose of 20 mg per day. She had joint pain, cognitive problems, hot flashes and she developed severe insomnia and energy depletion secondary to tamoxifen therapy. She was not a happy camper. The side effects from tamoxifen made her stop all therapies. She chose to do nothing rather than live in misery caused by the medication. She became motivated to seek modifications in her approach. This was what she sought in her first appointment with me.

I have observed that tamoxifen is a cumulative medication, that is, it tends to build up beyond minimum effective therapeutic doses the longer one takes it. This excessive build up together with limited ability in some patients to detoxify the drug is behind side effects that can make the drug intolerable. I have also discovered that patients can often achieve effective results by using pulsing-microdose with full-dose tamoxifen. The process of building up to a therapeutic threshold over two weeks then taking the full dose several times a week rather than daily while using microdoses of the drug on off days can be an effective therapy while greatly reducing side effects. It allows the

WHAT ARE CA-15-3 AND CA-27-29?

CA-15-3 and CA-27-29 are enzymes that become elevated due to inflammation from cancer growth. They are used as markers to determine whether a patient's cancer has returned.

patient to gain a modicum of control over life-disrupting side effects of estrogen withdrawal caused by medications yet still stay within a minimally effective therapeutic threshold. In short, not burdening the liver as much by reducing accumulations of medication in the body. This build up is what is often responsible for side effects, which cause patients to give up this potentially effective avenue of cancer-slowing therapy.

Barbara started to take 25 mg of tamoxifen twice a week. She also placed 25 mg of tamoxifen in 15 percent alcohol and water solution. Barbara took 60 drops of this solution twice a day. In this way, instead of 25 mg daily, she was taking 1.66 mg per day, five days per week and 25 mg, two days per week.

At the same time, Barbara's oncologist monitored her response and cancer markers CA 15-3 and CA 27-29 as well as her estradiol blood levels over the next month. Her estrogen levels remained below 12, and her symptoms completely disappeared. Her cancer markers remained at the levels they were prior to starting the pulse-microdosing.

Barbara remained on the pulse-microdose of tamoxifen and her condition remained stable. She had an annual MRI and ultrasound, but she did not use mammograms yearly since they were ineffective at discovering her cancer. She also continued to measure her CA 15-3 levels every six months, performed regular self-breast exams and monitored quantities of circulating tumor cells through blood testing with her oncologist.

In addition to addressing the first goal of containing the cancer over time, Barbara worked regularly on the second and third goals of detoxification and elimination. I gave Barbara a detoxification schedule that included colon cleansing, liver cleansing, lymphatic cleansing through sweating and sauna, a juicing protocol and diet to reduce inflammation and to help the process of cleansing, especially the liver. Her diet and life style became her most effective strategies. She also took I3C, a concentrate from broccoli which aids in processing estrogens and androgens safely.

We also performed a thorough exam of her teeth and reviewed dental fillings and crowns. Barbara went to a dentist to check for silent infections from stressed gums and teeth including root canals. Silent infections under root-canaled teeth can place a heavy burden on an already stressed immune system. Hidden burdens or focal disturbances are blockages that often obstruct the body's healing capacity. Any area of the body that has chronic inflammation such as chronic subclinical appendicitis, a chronic infection in a tooth or a chronic scar that hasn't properly healed can become a focal disturbance and become a roadblock to health or even cause more disease. It's very important to address those focal blockages as part of the detoxification elimination process. By removing roadblocks from the body's self-healing capacity we can unburden healing potentials. On the other hand, if a cancer patient has a mouthful of silver mercury amalgams it is important not to jump in too aggressively thus overwhelming a person's capacity to detoxify. This process must be individualized for every patient. When a person is already dealing with a flood you don't want to raise the water level even higher at the wrong time. This means that caution and care are foremost when dealing with a very serious condition. The process of chelating or detoxifying heavy metals at the same time that you're trying to regulate a cancer can actually decrease the ability of the immune system to work and put an extra burden and stress on the body. *The basic rule is: the sicker a person, the more carefully one should proceed with detoxification—easy does it over time.*

I asked Barbara to implement some dietary changes that included alkalizing, low-sugar and low carbohydrate, anti-inflammatory foods. In some cases, I will ask cancer patients to follow a vegetarian diet because it has an alkalinizing effect on the body; however, this is certainly not right for every constitution or person. Cancer cells both help create as well as thrive in acidic, low-oxygen microenvironments. Alkalinizing the body can assist with controlling the cancer, relaxing some of the toxic burden created by the cancer as well as the treatment of cancer with extremely acidifying chemo therapies. The burden on the kidneys, liver and lymphatic system is barely thought of in oncology except under extreme pathological conditions. When these organ systems are considered it is usually an afterthought. Unless the iceberg is above the pathology water line there is little consideration of the extreme effects from chemotherapy on acidosis and dehydration. One effective means of achieving alkalinity is through juicing of green vegetables including cruciferous vegetables such a broccoli, cauliflower and kale. One simple yet underemployed strategy for reducing the effects of chemotherapy on the body is to give hydration with normal physiologic saline after each treatment session.

There is no one diet for every patient with cancer any more than there's one diet for every human being. We have different constitutions, we have different digestive capacities, we have different needs. Diets, detoxification and alkalization strategies have to be individualized. When we grab a handle to slow down a cancer we must do so with careful observation of each person's response to a range of different variables. In other words, engage strategies then observe closely and respond appropriately and effectively to what is before us. There are multiple natural therapies that can be useful in helping to slow cancer expression and also reduce chemical side effects on the normal cells of the body. There are few silver bullets for cancer, especially a potentially metastasizing cancer like breast cancer or prostate cancer or any adenocarcinoma for that matter. These cancers are inherently prone to adapt, become aggressive, then metastasize.

When Barbara first came to me six months after her lumpectomy, I also noticed that the scar on her breast from surgery was still slightly tender, red and inflamed. I could feel there was an unresolved blood clot known as a hematoma below the surface of the surgical site. Hematomas are quite common after surgery, especially breast lumpectomies. Barbara also had significant scarring due to a post-surgical inflammatory process. She also had significant internal scars called adhesions so it was painful when she stretched her arm. Her range of motion was about 30 percent less than normal in trying to raise her arm above her head. I injected the scar tissue superficially with lidocaine and a homeopathic remedy for injections called Traumeel® using an acupuncture-sized, 30-gauge needle. I performed this simple and quick procedure because the scar is none other than a disrupted healing process. After two weeks Barbara noticed that the range of motion of her arm had improved dramatically. Also, the discomfort around the scar was gone and the tissue felt softer and looked less inflamed. Areas of scar tissue are often tissue where tumors return. In part, this is because the scar lacks adequate circulation, lymphatic drainage and immune function. In Barbara's case the scar tissue was both inflamed and hypoxic—ripe territory for cancer to return.

Surgeons cannot remove every cancer cell no matter how clean the margin in a lumpectomy or a mastectomy. Even though there are no traceable visual or palpable signs of its presence, there will always remain a few local cancer cells and many more circulating tumor cells. Not that these will necessarily become tumors in the future—how many seeds in nature actually become trees? Yet, you cannot remove all the cancer mechanically. Consequently, cancer cells can remain at the site of the scar tissue and, once cancer reignites or reinvents itself, can and does often contribute to the return of tumors both locally and at distant locations from the original cancerous lump.

A New Way to Monitor Barbara's Progress

In 2004, I began using a new test to monitor whether or not Barbara's cancer had returned. The CA 15-3 and CA 27-29 cancer markers that I had been using are shadow dancers with cancer—they're not actually a direct measurement of cancer. They are inflammatory enzyme tests that may or may not be useful for monitoring cancer. The test I started using in 2004, which measures circulating tumor cell counts, is a much more specific way to identify the potential presence or absence as well as state of cancer expression in the body. The circulating tumor cell count is a direct look at what's going on with the cancer rather than a shadow dance with an enzyme that shows up due to inflammation from cancer growth.

Circulating tumor cells are important because these types of cancers circulate in the blood stream. They are systemic. Once the genie's out of the bag that person who has cancer is always going to have circulating tumor cells the rest of his or her life even if a lump never comes back in any organ of the body. By isolating those circulating tumor cells and identifying how many there are per ml of blood, it is possible to determine whether therapies are effective and if cancer metastasic potential is rising. This test is based upon the number of cancer cells present in the patient's blood as well as upon whether there's been a return of an aggressive cancer profile. Briefly stated, the test is interpreted upon whether the number of circulating tumor cells are going up or down over time. That is a quantifiable measurement. We're all fighting cancer but we do not have circulating tumor cells in our blood unless there is cancer present. Yet, the genetics of those circulating tumor cells allow oncologists and patients to get a biopsy, whereas tumor biopsies in organs are often very invasive and dangerous.

You can perform a genetic fingerprint on the population of isolated circulating tumor cells and look at the entire mutanome. It seems reasonable to perform the circulating tumor cell blood test at regular intervals on every cancer patient who has a potentially metastasizing cancer. That fingerprint shows you which genes are overexpressed and how overexpressed they are and what their function is, whether they're inflammatory, whether they represent fast metabolism, if they represent mutational metabolism, if they represent blood vessel growth metabolism, if they indicate resistance metabolism, if they represent blockage of apoptosis metabolism or if the cancer is hormone activated. And all those factors are part of the software of cancers. Once the exact overall fingerprint of that software is obtained, you can test that population of cells for what therapies may be most effective: chemotherapies, directed monoclonal antibodies, targeted therapies, and in some cases hormone-blocking therapies. This type of testing can also help determine which nutrients are most effective. It is one method of developing a rational therapeutic strategy.

Changing Barbara's Game Plan

Barbara remained on the microdose of tamoxifen until 2008. At this point, concerned about the long-term effects of tamoxifen, she talked to her oncologist about ceasing the drug. I remembered she had osteopenia (thinning bones). There is a medication called raloxifene (Evista®) that also has been found to block estrogen receptors. We switched her over to raloxifene. For a couple of weeks, she took the full dose of 60 mg daily, but her menopausal symptoms returned. She suffered from brain fog, emotional volatility, sore joints, hot flashes, insomnia and overall discomfort, which indicates that the drug affects estrogen receptors since it threw her into the same symptoms as tamoxifen or an aromatase inhibitor would have.

Barbara implemented a similar pulse-microdosing strategy as she had done with tamoxifen. She took the full dose of 60 mg raloxifene two days per week. She also made a dilution of one, 60 mg raloxifene in a 2-ounce bottle of a homeopathic remedy for the immune system. This amounted to 2 mgs per day of raloxifene for five days per week rather than 60 mgs per day. In other words, she did pulse therapy at full dose for two days to maintain that threshold level and the microdosing on days that she didn't take the full pill. By doing this, her menopausal symptoms disappeared.

From 2008 to 2014, she continued to use the pulse/microdosing regimen while monitoring her circulating tumor cells and cancer markers three times per year. She took extra vitamin D for her osteopenia, she exercised and maintained a good diet.

In 2014, she wanted to stop taking the raloxifene. Her cancer had been gone for 15 years and her CA 15-3 was normal. Her circulating tumor cell count was a little elevated, but not enough to warrant concern. I suggested that she consult with her oncologist and if she stopped taking the raloxifene, get an MRI within three months.

Barbara stopped taking the raloxifene. Within eight weeks of stopping the drug she noticed a swelling in her left breast in a different area than where the original tumor had been: at 2 o'clock in the upper outer quadrant of the breast. An MRI revealed the presence of another tumor.

Barbara's original surgical oncologist performed a biopsy and a lumpectomy and found that the tumor was the same exact cancer as before: an infiltrating ductal carcinoma in situ. It was estrogen 100 percent positive, progesterone 30 percent positive and HER2/neu negative.

The oncologist recommended chemotherapy and radiation, which Barbara refused. She preferred to do watchful waiting and follow up consults. Her oncologist agreed to this strategy, partly because she knew Barbara had a 15-year plus history of adenocarcinoma and she had been well maintained during that time.

We placed Barbara back on the pulse-microdosing of raloxifene and there has been no expression of her cancer since that time.

Fear-Based Medicine

Barbara's case serves as an example that individualizing care can open up and expand to opportunities for patients. Cancer patients and their families who act out of information rather than fear can make better decisions about their care. It's important for people to be educated about what it is they're dealing with as well as the latest science and targeted trials. No one has a handle on absolute good outcome in cancer. No one. It is many, many diseases rather than one. It's a molecular, oncogenetic, mutational disease and arguably it is an environmental illness. But it occurs in individuals, and until we get to the point of at least attempting individualized molecular analysis and targeting the immune system as much as the tumor we're not going to optimize outcomes. We're treating that ship like it's a Chinese boat with rice when many times it's not. And once it gets into port if we haven't analyzed it correctly we can find ourselves in troubled waters.

Always ask: "If I do the treatment you're prescribing by what percentage will it lower cancer's return? How does that compare to not doing the therapy? Are there other alternatives? What are the chances of side effects short term and long term?" Since you're dealing with statistical analysis you might as well know the numbers. Having information, putting different opinions on the table then carefully considering these will allow a sense of peace with the path chosen. Make decisions out of information rather than fear. No matter what choice is made.

I'm interested in prevention, I'm interested in understanding and in sharing the understanding of what a person is actually dealing with when a cancer emerges in their life or the life of family and friends. I'm interested in greater access to science, in monitoring blood for circulating cancer stem cells, epigenetic protein expressions and nutritional protocols, lifestyle and environmental approaches to prevention, early detection and chronic management. This includes not only traditional chemotherapy, radiation and surgery, but also innovative autologous tumor cell vaccine therapies, targeted therapies such as multiple low dose and chronometric monoclonal antibodies, amino acid targeted therapies and other innovations to put ankle weights on the ability of a cancer to grow thus allowing a person to live with rather than for cancer.

WHAT IS AUTOLOGOUS TUMOR CELL VACCINE THERAPY?

An autologous tumor cell vaccine is made by isolating tumor cells from an individual and using those tumor cells to create a vaccine in cell culture. The vaccine is then administered to the same person who provided those tumor cells.

Instead of dropping atomic bombs on tumors thus killing the tumor and all too often the patient, we should treat cancer as the chronic illness it is. A small number of cancer cells often exist years before a trauma, a shock, a chronic degenerative inflammation, an injury or an immune-suppressing life event allows and ignites a small number of mutated cells that then emerge as a lump of 400 to 700 million cells before being discovered. We can and must do better. We certainly know better at this point in time.

The incredible breakthroughs and innovations in cancer research light the way, yet are all too often ten to fifteen years ahead of clinical applications and public access. Times are changing, yet future promises do nothing to help address the needs of a person suffering from the immediate need for innovation and individualization of treatment. I do believe we'll have much better outcomes with various cancer-controlling therapies in the future, but these will not eliminate the environmental toxicities that are actually responsible for cell mutations. Cancer therapies do not eliminate stress itself or emotional trauma any more than human pollution, war or environmental degradations, so cancer is not going to go away. But hopefully our understanding of the bigger picture will improve and our ability to manage the expression of cancer over time will be both more benign and more effective.

CHAPTER 3

A Brief Personal History—Making It Real

Anyone who practices healing arts has their own life experiences to draw from. We have all experienced life's challenges from the first breath we take to survive to our last breath. Stress in its various forms is inherent in life. In my own case, I was brought into the world with high forceps delivery, which traumatized my nervous system resulting in severe colic for most of my first year of life. I almost didn't survive. I tenaciously and tenuously clung to life. I couldn't keep anything in. My mother couldn't produce enough breast milk, so she was encouraged to give me formula, cow's milk and soy-based formulas. I reacted adversely to everything they tried. Eventually, an old family doctor told my mother to try goat's milk. Finally, I thrived and survived that turbulent beginning. Luckily, after the near-death experience of my first year, I've enjoyed a healthy childhood and adult life, hard head and all.

Over the years I've encountered various traditional cultural concepts for physical, emotional and spiritual challenges. One that has stayed with me and that I tell my very ill patients about is called "Nierica," the Quichol Indian concept for a doorway of the spirit. Here is a brief personal description of Nierica I shared in a letter to a close friend who was very ill:

"This time has been a Nierica for you to be sure—coyote/ Nierica time. The Quichol word for spiritual opening or divine doorway is Nierica. A Nierica can be a portal covered with roses, full of thorns, on fire, scalding, burning, traumatic. To stand in the doorway and not pass through can be excruciating. Sometimes we have to wait at the threshold for the door to open wide. Once we have passed through the portal we can live life with a fullness, appreciation and gratitude, with humility that comes from the fire walk of passing through even though we have fear, trepidation, despair and deep depression or sadness about the process. It is a spiritual cleansing, a letting go, a surrendering to greater intelligence than our own ignorant willfulness, and it can be most difficult. The soul walks with the body, the higher-self watches and guides, the divine self exalts in the passionate transformation of the physical body as we increase in consciousness. You're waiting at the threshold at this time. I've been there before in life. I know how it feels personally to have to pass through; I've held many hands and encouraged many souls in their own journey through the portal. Now it's your turn again. Let go of fear. There's impatience perhaps but let fear's cold hand go. It's just a matter of time. Ask for guidance and protection. It's just a matter of time. You'll pass through the doorway then fear will have no hold on you, no matter what the outcome. Take care my friend,"

When patients come to me who are facing life and death struggles I try to let them know that they are in a Nierica

Doorway, one that will transform them, one that they will overcome only by surrendering to and passing through, one that is informing them about how precious life is and about what is really important in life. My patients are my teachers; their struggle gives me perspective on my own day-to-day concerns. Standing at the Nierica doorway, then eventually passing through it transforms us, makes us more appreciative of life and gives us compassion for the suffering of others.

My older brother Tom died at age 54 of colon cancer. When Tom was in his last month of life, when surgery and medical treatments had not only failed to help him, but devitalized him to within an inch of losing life, he wrote a beautiful little piece for family and friends called, *"Death as an Ally."* What Tom wrote about was how the knowledge of imminent death had taught him to live life to the fullest. If he didn't want to be around somebody he'd just say it. He became aware of his own needs and if he didn't want to do something he wouldn't do it and if he wanted to enjoy something he'd enjoy it in the present. He lived every moment to the fullest and shared his dying with family and friends. He shared with all of us how much the process of dying is a form of birthing—difficult, often painful, heart opening and certain.

We live with the paradox of feeling most alive when we realize the inevitability of dying, and living life devoid of expressing ourselves or being un-self aware is surely just a form of living death.

I remember one morning, when I was about four or five years old, my father was doubled over in pain on the living room couch. He had been a GI in World War II in Europe and then, several months after returning from Europe, was on a convoy headed for the invasion of Japan. Suddenly, on his 31st birthday, August 6, 1945, when they were mid Pacific, the ships turned around and headed back for the States. They were told the War was over because of a single bomb. My dad told me that no one believed that the War was over until they actually did turn around and headed for home. My dad arrived home to San Francisco to my mother and my older brother Tom, to his own mother, his brothers and sisters, aunts and uncles, cousins and friends. He put on a tie and went back to work just like thousands of other veterans.

But this morning, my dad couldn't get up off the couch. He was in so much pain he could barely breathe. My mother called our family doctor, Dr. Tom Sawyer, who promptly came over to our house. Dr. Sawyer sat in a chair next to my dad with his hand gently resting on my dad's shoulder, softly speaking to him and listening as my dad responded. I remember going in and out of their space the way only a child can, without being noticed, not really understanding what was being said but noticing the gentle energy between them. Suddenly, my dad just stood up, straightened his tie, put on his coat and went to work. My mom was happy but astonished. After my dad had left she asked Dr. Sawyer what he had done, why my dad had been able to just spring up as though nothing had been wrong and go off to face the day. Dr. Sawyer responded, "Oh, we just talked about the War a little."

Post-traumatic stress hadn't been defined yet, but the body doesn't need a diagnosis to feel the pain and the stress after returning from war or other trauma and challenges of life. Sometimes just acknowledging the pain and stress is enough to turn a downward, ailing spiral into an upward, healing spiral.

Even though nothing has really changed at the moment, the simple act of listening, really listening to our self or having the ear of a compassionate person, really listening, is enough to turn us around. The healing begins, holographically spreading throughout the body, influencing the way we think and, transforming negative feelings into positive, life-regenerating patterns of experience.

It's when we ignore the road signs which say, *"Go Slow, Dangerous Curves,"* when we simply throw a blanket over the sign and proceed full speed ahead, that we go over the cliff full speed, wondering how things could have gone wrong.

Sometimes, when people go to see their doctor, they come in complaining about their elbow, but the elbow is really just the tip of the iceberg. To illustrate this point, I want to tell you about a dream I had once.

My Dream of Death as My Patient

When I worked in NYC with Dr. Robert Atkins during the 1980s and the nurses were too busy, I would walk out to the waiting room to lead my next patient down the hall and into my office. I once had a dream wherein I went out to the waiting room and it was like Grand Central Station. There were thousands of people there waiting. I noticed a little elderly gentleman sitting quietly in the corner. I took a chart and said, "Next please," then turned and walked down the hall. As I got to my office I turned to see the old man walking down the hall behind me. He came in and sat down in front of me. I looked into his face and saw deep lines and pain in his eyes. I glanced at his medical chart. The name printed on the label was *"Death."*

So I asked Death what his problem was. He proceeded to begin complaining, "My elbow hurts, my arm hurts, my feet hurt, I'm aching all over, I have no energy, I can't sleep, I'm depressed, and I hate my job. Nobody likes me, nobody wants me to come over. I can't eat, I can't stop thinking about eating, I can't sleep. I just can't go on being Death anymore."

As I sat listening to Death's litany of pains and sorrows I realized that when people go to the doctor it's often because when we feel sick we also feel mortal. We feel vulnerable and sometimes we feel afraid. Going to the doctor reassures us that we're not going to die, yet. Then, I also realized that a truckload of medicine or healing nutrients does no good so long as the soul is holding an empty cup.

After listening to Death, I gazed at him sitting before me, crinkled up and hunched over. I said to him, "Why are you so miserable being yourself?"

Death tilted his head, leaned forward, looking at me with hollowed, yellowed eyes, and said, "Why am I so miserable being myself? I'm miserable 'cause it's so hard living when you're dead."

The self-healing body whether it succeeds in healing or fails, never gives up. It's in our own hands whether we block its path or help by removing obstacles to health.

An Anatomy Lesson in the Dance of Life

I have been blessed with two children, my daughter Ariana and my son Ciancarlo. When Ariana was a little over three years old, I started taking her to ballet performances at the San Francisco opera house. She loved the music, the costumes and the dance so much that she would sit transfixed through the entire performance. She would only get up during intermission, then be right back in her seat as the second act began. Once I took Ariana to see *Giselle*. We had seats on the left balcony just a few feet from the stage. The first act went by, the gypsies dancing, the colorful pageantry of the costumes delighting Ariana as usual. After getting settled into our seats for the second act, the colors and tone of the ballet changed. Giselle had died and became a wood nymph, her prince came looking for her in the forest and they danced together, but the prince couldn't see Giselle. At one point in his grand dance the prince, in skin-colored tights, landed stage left just a few feet from where Ariana and I sat. The prince stood there before us, arms outstretched to the side, plied and still. There was a pause in the music and a brief silence. Suddenly Ariana said for all to hear, "Papa, how come that prince doesn't have a penis?" I sunk down deep into my seat as muffled snickers rose from the orchestra pit. The poor prince glanced down very briefly to check himself and then leapt back into the dance. Sometimes, no matter what, we just have to keep dancing.

About Quacks

One evening around 1986, I met a retired, 94-year-old physician at a gathering in Brooklyn. We started up a conversation and he said to me, "Oh, so you're in medicine. So where do you practice?"

I answered, "With Dr. Robert Atkins at his alternative medical center."

The old physician's eyes widened as he said with a little grin, "Oh, so you're a quack."

I laughed, then said, "Do you know where the word quack comes from? It comes from quacksilver/quicksilver, an archaic word for mercury. They used to use mercury for treating syphilis."

He said, "Oh, yes. I treated many patients with mercury. In fact, we had a saying, 'One night with Venus and the rest of your life with Mercury.'"

"Oh, so you're the quack," I said, smiling and pointing a finger. He laughed and we laughed together.

 Take Home Points

- I tell my patients who are battling life and death struggles that they must step through what the Quichol Indians call a Nierica Doorway. It is only by surrendering to and passing through this metaphorical doorway that you will be informed about how precious life is and about what is really important to you.

- Sometimes, especially in the case of mental challenges such as post-traumatic stress disorder, just acknowledging your pain and stress is enough to turn a downward, ailing spiral into an upward, healing spiral. Even though nothing has really changed at the moment, the simple act of listening, really listening to our self or having the ear of a compassionate person, really listening, is enough to turn us around.

- It's in your own hands whether you block your self-healing body's path or help by removing obstacles to health.

CHAPTER 4

How Complex Systems Create the Unexpected

Now that I have shown you how we are part of bigger and smaller realities, both fractal and holographic, and how healing emerges from these different quantum levels, I want to talk a bit about complex systems. All humans are incredibly complex made up of different complex systems smaller and larger.

Physicians, clinicians and practitioners of medical arts must incorporate disciplines from many sciences, cultures and traditions every day. In order to fully understand any complex system from a vernal pond to a governmental bureaucracy, subatomic particle physics to cosmology, sandwiches to stem cells, evolutionary diversity to the digestion of our lunch, many disciplines or ways of knowing must be used simultaneously.

Emergence is a natural consequence of a system achieving a critical mass of complexity giving rise to another level of phenomena. For example, thought itself is an emergence from the complexity of our holographic neuroanatomy proceeded by a billion years of life on the planet which itself emerged from the complexity of a timeless, evolving universe. The macro cosmos not only reflects the micro cosmos but one creates or emerges from

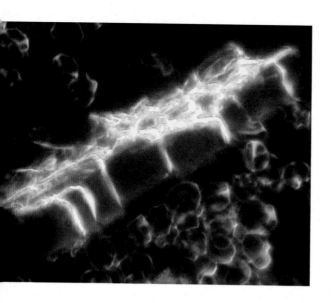

the other. The quest for the ultimate elemental particle has brought us to strings or resonance from which emerges at least eleven dimensions of reality. Ultimately all things cosmic to microcosmic begin and end with resonance and harmonics. The mathematical expression of these phenomena of emergence in Nature is found in fractal geometry, which is the geometry of a holographic universe. This is why, when someone says to me, "How can you occasionally see distressed organs and structures of the body in dark field examination of blood," I always answer the same way, "Why not, it's part of the same Universe we all inhabit and that Universe is both fractal and holographic."

Complex Systems

Complex systems can be defined as an accumulation of diversity interacting to create new emerging phenomena known as "phase transition" in science. Think about one molecule of water verses an ocean of H_2O molecules and what emerges from that complexity.

Now here's a definition of emergence: increasing complexity creates the emergence of new properties not previously present in either a single member or the group. The emergence is a higher level of complexity created as a natural consequence of any complex system. In short, "the unexpected happens."

Achieving a critical mass of complexity, any complex system produces unexpected phenomena. Think of a drop of water verses an ocean and then, clouds, storms, hurricanes, currents, weather patterns, fog, waves, tsunamis and wind patterns not to mention emergent life forms. There's nothing very complicated about a single water molecule—H_2O. Then place 10 to the ten gigazillion of these simple molecules together. Suddenly you've got a substance that shimmers and gurgles and sloshes. Those zillions of molecules have collectively acquired a property—liquidity. Liquidity is emergent. Emergent properties produce emergent

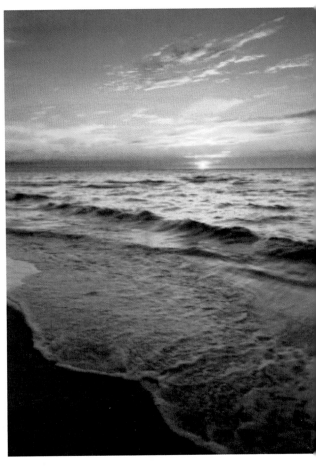

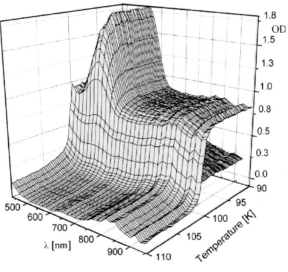

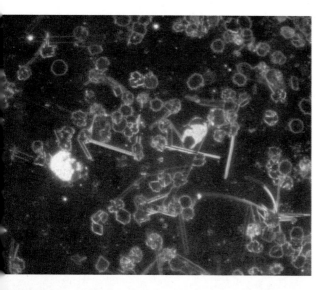

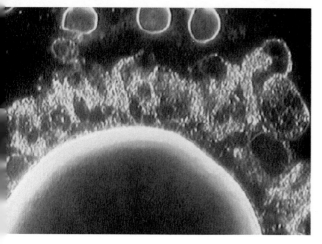

behaviors in much the same way.

Cool liquid water molecules slow down a bit and at 32 degrees F they will suddenly quit tumbling over one another at random. Instead, they will undergo "phase transition"—there's that term again—and the phase transition caused by freezing temperatures locks the water molecules into the orderly crystalline array known as ice. Or, if you were to go in the other direction, and heat the liquid, those same tumbling water molecules will suddenly fly apart and undergo a phase transition into water vapor. Neither phase would have any meaning for a single molecule. In a complex system of water molecules, however, emergence occurs regularly. These examples can be extended to other complex systems, for example human blood, or as a model for understanding cancers.

Red blood cells, white blood cells, platelets, fibrinogen, plasma cytokines, nutrients, proteins and fats, antibodies, all that is contained in our blood undergo phase transitions as various cells age. The still living blood cells reorganize themselves as vitality and oxygen supply change. When a drop of blood is placed on a glass slide and viewed under a dark field microscope, which allows the sample to be observed in a still living state without heating it up, one can observe emergent holographic crystallizations as well as an overall emergent self-reorganization of

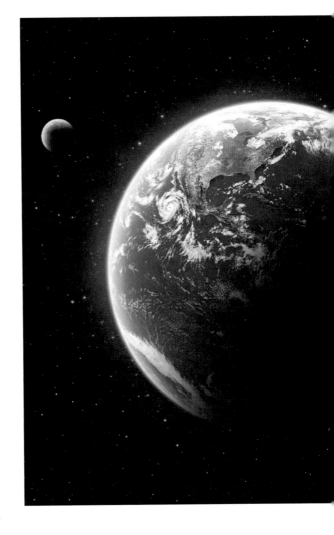

the blood cells under stress conditions outside the body.

In addition to all that is considered normal blood complexity, there are yet more complex layers of reality emerging within blood. Perceiving emergent patterns by observation over time is essential to understanding the myriad phenomena occurring in the complex system of blood. The degree of order or chaos seen over time in blood can be predictive of the overall health of the whole organism. Blood reflects inherent fractal phenomena since it is part of the fractal body and fractal holographic universe.

Life Systems

Life systems are emergent, the product of DNA, carbon chain molecules, protein molecules and myriad other kinds of molecules all obeying self-organizing laws of chemical biology and physics. The mind is an emergent property, the product of billions of specialized neurons obeying the biological laws of the living organism yet also creating a new, emergent holography, which we humans call "the self." It has also been said that we are essentially spiritual beings, but we are in a physical body and so that spirit emerges in this life from the physical complexity of our Earth based life form. Many traditional cultures extend this emergent spirit concept to all things living and inanimate, including the living Earth planet, known to ancient Greeks as Gaia

Other examples of emergent patterns include weather. Take water vapor over the Gulf of Mexico interacting with sunlight and wind and organizing itself into an emergent structure known as a hurricane. In fact, at each level of complexity entirely new properties appear, and at each stage, entirely new laws, concepts and collective self-organizations occur.

Once certain molecules, substrates and catalysts occurred, the emergence of life forms became inevitable. Rather than a random, freak accident of nature, life appears as an inexorable manifestation of emergence in the cosmos when a critical degree of complexity of elements and molecules coalesce. Complexity, in other words, is the science of emergence.

So the story of life is the story of accident and happenstance, but also the story of self-ordering complexity, a kind of deep, inner creativity that is woven into the very fabric of nature. Great emerging areas in science are ones involving many disciplines. Back in 1932, the physicist who discovered the positron—the antimatter version of the electron—declared: "The rest is chemistry." There has been a prevalent belief among scientists that fundamental particles are the only thing that's worth studying and that everything else could be predicted if you only had a big enough computer. But the ability to reduce everything to simple fundamental laws does not imply the ability to start from those laws and reconstruct the universe. In fact, the more the elemental particle physicists tell us about the nature of the fundamental laws the less relevance they seem to have to the very real problems of the rest of science, much less society.

The mathematical expression of a fundamentally holographic Universe is fractal geometry. Once there is an accumulated diversity, a system goes through a phase transition where there is an enormous proliferation of things at that level. Scale and complexity create what is called an emergent phenomenon. This is the appearance of a characteristic or a quality that emerges unexpectedly from a complex system. The proliferation of members of a complex system produce things at more complex and higher energetic levels then the individual components of the system alone could produce. For example:

Matter:

Solid => phase transition => fluid=> phase transition=> gas

Life Systems:

chaos=> self-organization=> living systems=> stasis => death=> new life =>

The rules of life are the only rules that provide enough stability to store information and enough fluidity to send signals over arbitrary distances. These rules sit right in phase transition at the edge of chaos. They not only live on the edge but they are always in danger of dropping off into too much order or too much chaos.

Evolution is a process of life learning how to adapt to more and more of its own limitations and constraints so that it has a better chance of survival. These rules apply to phase transitions but hold true on our level of reality as well in everything from social systems to economies to living cells. Life depends to a great degree on its ability to process information. Cells do not just respond like a rock to forces applied to them, but rather like a flock of birds in flight. Their reaction to constraint or freedom, nourishment or trauma and inflammation is complex. Longevity of a blood sample reflects the ability of cells to maintain vitality. Inflammation and the rapid disintegration of cells reflect stress and lack of vitality moving toward chaotic conditions then stasis. Free radicals and oxidized, low-energy or acidic states lead to the chaotic breakdown of cell organization, and ultimately to death. The mysterious something that makes life and mind possible is a balance between the forces of order and of disorder.

Evolution thrives in systems with a bottom up organization, which gives rise to flexibility, but at the same time evolution has to focus the bottom up approach in a way that doesn't destroy the organization. There has to be a hierarchy of control with information flowing from the bottom up as well as from the top down. This is a holographic system. This reality of organization in the Cosmos essentially represents an alteration of the second Law of Thermodynamics—not only is entropy or loss of energy and organization inevitable, so is self-organization in this Universe.

Fractal patterns appear ubiquitously in nature. They occur on the level of the distribution of galaxies throughout the Cosmos, geometric shapes mirrored macro and microscopically, the shape of coastlines or the edge of a blood slide, clouds, waves and all patterns in nature. A fractal is a geometric shape that can be separated into parts, each of which is a reduced scale version of the whole, i.e. a hologram. String harmonics, sub-atomic particles, atoms, molecules, living cells, multi-cellular organisms, cultures, ecosystems, planets, solar systems, galaxies, galactic clusters, and universes. One form emerges from another, living cells, organisms, cultures, planets, solar systems. Ultimately, all returns to harmonics, and each new emerging level of organization is alive in the same sense as the component parts that create it.

Back to the Mandala

Now I'd like to focus once again upon what I'm calling the Holosystemic Mandala. This Mandala reflects in colors the ground up and top down complexity of our bodies. Each of us comes into this world in a space suit we call the human body but no one ever enters this life with an operator's manual, not as far as I've ever observed at least. Over the next few pages are illustrations of this Holosystemic Mandala, an owner's guide for the human body.

THE HOLOSYSTEMIC MANDALA
An Owner's Guide For The Human Body

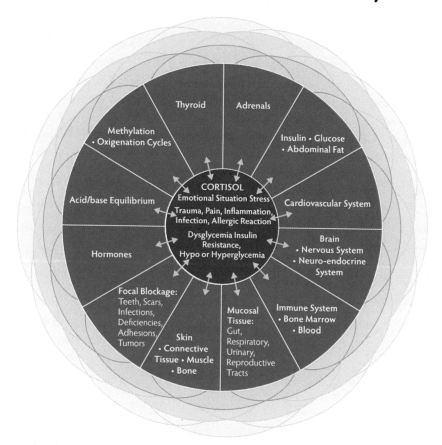

Blue—The Optimal Ideal State

Notice that the center of the mandala is cortisol. The reason cortisol is the key to understanding our complex and self-healing body is because over the past four and a half billion years all emergent life forms of Earth have struggled to survive. Cortisol is your emergent survival hormone. It is our body's normal physiologic response to sudden, on-going or increasing stresses of living on planet Earth. Cortisol is our survival response hormone. Here, once again, are the three primary forms of stress:

a.) Emotional /situational stress

b.) Physical Stress including: trauma, pain, inflammation, infection, allergic reaction

c.) Physiologic Stress: dysglycemia (hypo or hyperglycemia: low or high blood sugar)

Our body translates all forms of stress into cortisol. So, from first breath until our last, stress is inherent in life. And from first breath until last cortisol is present to help us survive. The blue mandala of perfect health changes with the birthing process. We add in survival stress and now the mandala takes on the normal adaptive state of life, the mandala turns from blue to green.

THE HOLOSYSTEMIC MANDALA
An Owner's Guide For The Human Body

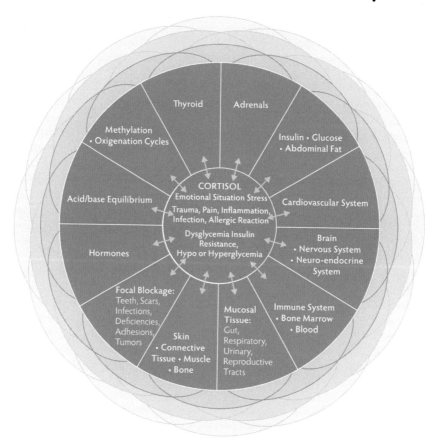

Green–Life Stress

Next, I'd like you to look around the center of the mandala. Notice that there are twelve systems surrounding the central survival hormone cortisol. Notice that there are two-way arrows between every system and cortisol. What I am demonstrating here is that the stress hormone cortisol has potential impacts on all body systems. Stress from the body's systems in turn can increase cortisol demand. This creates the potential for negative feedback loops between stress and the basic systems of our body. In other words, our body can get stuck in physiologic ruts, which then begin to interfere with function and even induce illness. The mandala is the soil out of which either health or what we call disease grows. The empty outer shells of the mandala represent what emerges from stresses and adaptations to various stresses in your body's entire ecosystem.

I don't want you to have to study all the details of the mandala. That's not important for this book, although the science behind these various connections is clear. The main point I want to make is that nothing in your body is isolated, every organ and system of the body communicates with every other part. Stress in its various forms and the body's response to stress—cortisol—potentially and practically interacts with your entire body. Over time, cumulative stresses increase your cortisol demand and may decrease the adrenals' capacity to keep up. This gradual accumulation of cortisol load creates negative feedback loops and ultimately degenerations in your weakest and most vulnerable systems. Depending on your genetics, life experiences and overall vitality, long-term cortisol demand will gradually erode your life force.

Long-term cortisol demand from various stress factors can begin to change the basic physiologic soil from which either health or chronic disease emerge. Problems often show up at the weakest link in the system. For one person it's insomnia, anxiety or depression, for another it's insulin resistance and then possibly diabetes, for another it may be a heart attack, and all too often, all of the above may occur at various times during our life or all at once like an avalanche.

Now I'm going to give you the color key to understanding the holosystemic mandala. I've shown you how the color **_blue represents perfect health_**. Then we add yellow and the mandala turns **_green, which represents a normal, healthy stress state_**. When pure **_yellow shows up there is an acute stress such as trauma, infection_** or maybe the baby is sick or you're going through a contentious divorce. Next, **_orange indicates a chronic, ongoing stress state_**. **_Red is a tipping point when chronic stresses evolve to where the body begins to lose its ability to self-correct_**. This could result in autoimmune illness or chronic degenerative conditions such as osteoarthritis, diabetes, psoriasis, etc. Finally, **_when violet emerges there is an advanced pathology such as a cancer or a heart attack_**.

Without getting into all the details and analysis, simply look at the color progression of the mandalas of a person who experiences stresses and imbalances with his or her body over time. These stresses eventually lead to a heart attack. This will show up as purple in the cardiovascular section of the mandala. Follow the colors. The exact symptoms and signs are not the point here although the changes in color give you clues about how this person might be feeling, no matter at what age or over what amount of time it takes for the progression to occur. For some it might be early in life, for others, scores of years into striving through life. Simply observe the color changes. When violet shows up observe how after being treated by emergency medical intervention and sent home, the person still has the same complex set of stresses which led to the heart attack to begin with. At this point, by changing diet, exercising, attitudes about sickness and health, taking adversity as an ally versus an opponent, reducing stresses and detoxifying, you can begin to reverse the sequence and move away from disease toward a more balanced state of health. The mandala reflects this over time. The following set of mandalas reflects one of many possible pathways, first towards and then away from heart attack.

THE HOLOSYSTEMIC MANDALA
An Owner's Guide For The Human Body

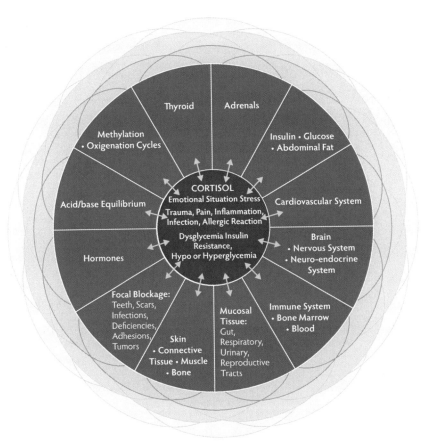

Perfect Health

THE HOLOSYSTEMIC MANDALA
An Owner's Guide For The Human Body

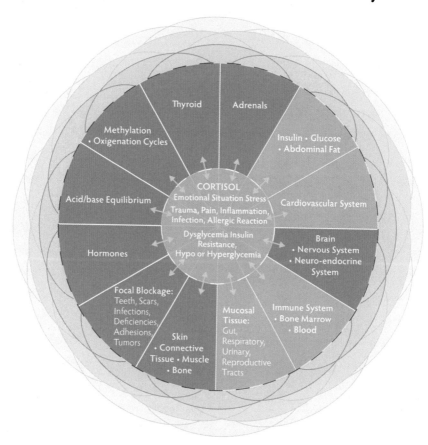

Normal Life Stress with Some Acute Stresses (Yellow)

THE HOLOSYSTEMIC MANDALA
An Owner's Guide For The Human Body

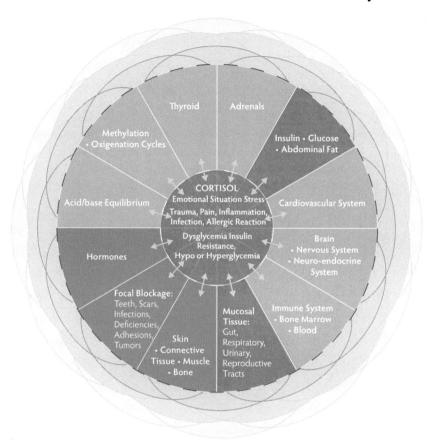

Increasing Chronic Stresses (Orange)
Loss of Vitality

THE HOLOSYSTEMIC MANDALA
An Owner's Guide For The Human Body

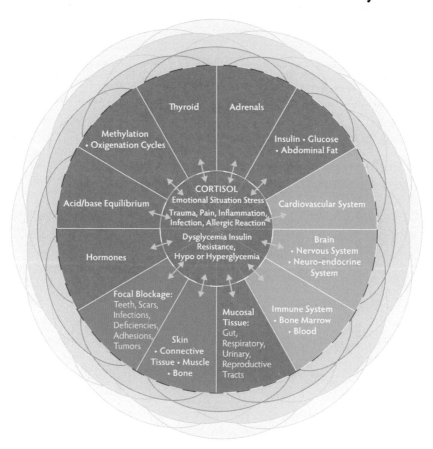

Serious Increase in Chronic Stress
Loss of vitality and chronic degeneration

THE HOLOSYSTEMIC MANDALA
An Owner's Guide For The Human Body

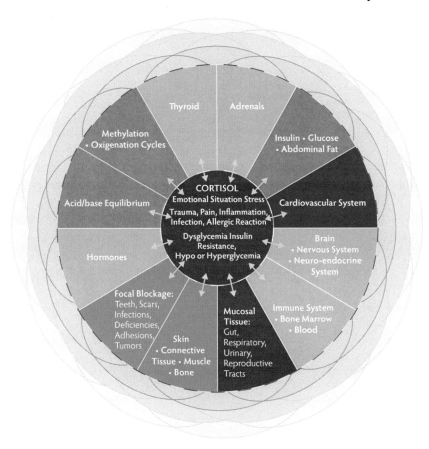

Emergence of Autoimmune Illness and Heart Pathology
Red–the body cannot reverse a condition on its own
Purple–an emerging pathology

THE HOLOSYSTEMIC MANDALA
An Owner's Guide For The Human Body

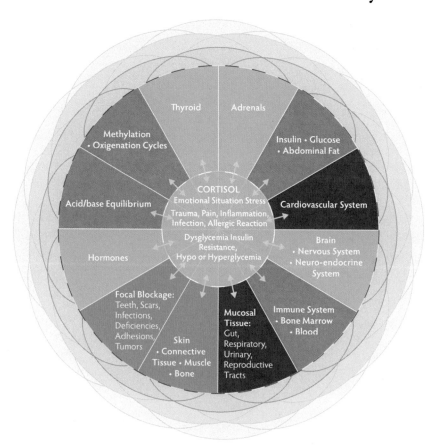

Stabilized Heart with Remaining Stress Vectors

THE HOLOSYSTEMIC MANDALA
An Owner's Guide For The Human Body

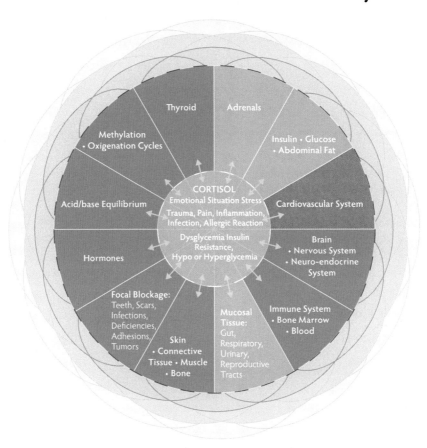

On the Way to Recovery, Old Symptoms Fade

THE HOLOSYSTEMIC MANDALA
An Owner's Guide For The Human Body

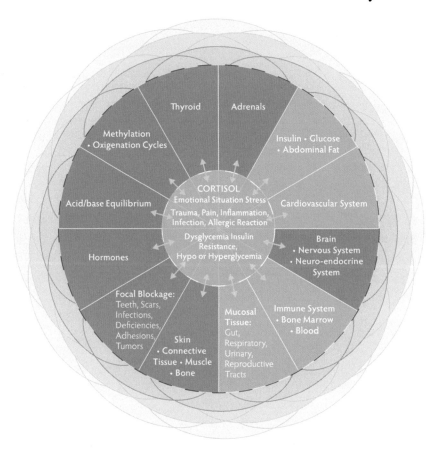

On the Way to Recovery, Vitality/Healing Potential Increases

THE HOLOSYSTEMIC MANDALA
An Owner's Guide For The Human Body

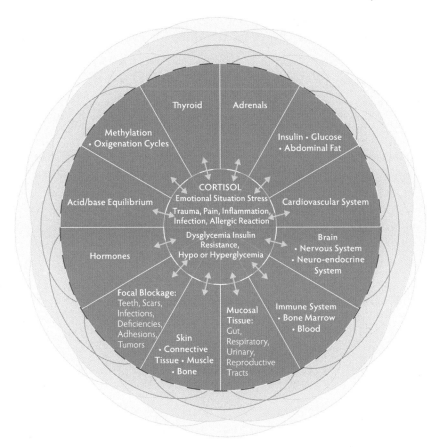

Healing–Nourishing All Systems

Now, how about your mandala? As I describe a real-life case, you can use the following blank mandala to fill in the colors of where your own system stresses have, are and might be showing. Or you can visit **www.biomedarts.com** to use my free Holosystemic Mandala App. Take your time and come back to this mandala as you read on. Your intuition, as well as your family and personal medical histories, are important clues for coloring in your own mandala.

THE HOLOSYSTEMIC MANDALA
An Owner's Guide For The Human Body

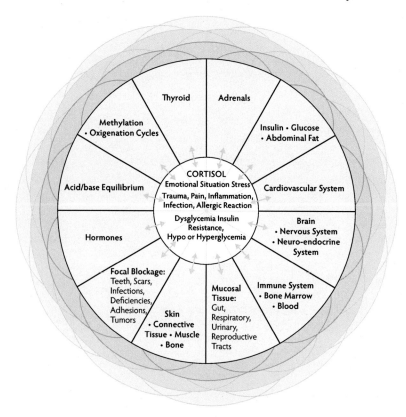

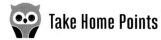 **Take Home Points**

- Cortisol is the key to understanding our complex and self-healing body.

- Our body translates all forms of stress into cortisol.

- The stress hormone cortisol has potential impacts on all of your body systems.

- By filling out your own Holosystemic Mandala, you can see how cortisol and stress are contributing to your own health conditions.

CHAPTER 5

Cortisol/Insulin Dynamics—An Epic Struggle

The dynamic relationship between insulin and glucose blood sugar levels is of critical importance in both the cause and prevention of disease. Maintaining proper glycemic control creates a fundamental solid foundation for enabling your body's self-healing potential. Glycemic imbalance, the interplay between low blood sugar or elevated blood sugar and the glucose regulating hormone insulin, can create a physiologic storm in which all systems and organs of the body are swamped. Of course, there are other endocrine factors involved as well such as glucagon, fat-based leptins, inflammatory cytokines and adipokines, epinephrine, norepinephrine, etc., but we'll mostly limit this discussion to basic insulin/cortisol dynamics.

The prime culprit in this epic struggle is what is now known as insulin resistance or metabolic syndrome. When you eat sugars, including high glycemic foods such as refined wheat (white breads), white rice, pastries, fruit juices, dried fruits, candy, soda and any packaged convenience food containing corn syrup sweeteners, you are putting paper on the fire so to speak. If you want to keep a fire burning and you just throw paper on it, you'll have to stand by all day tossing in paper just to keep the fire from burning out. In other words it takes a lot more work to keep the fire burning. Your glucose rises rapidly, the pancreatic beta cells secrete insulin and then your blood sugar drops, your energy sinks, your brain disengages, your vision might get blurry, your heart beat may become irregular or race and you feel overwhelmed and then get irritable or want to crawl into your shell. If you're the tough–it-out type, then you use your reserve fuel system via cortisol and push through. Over time the high cortisol demand diminishes the adrenal glands' capacity and vitality begins to wane. This hypoglycemic/cortisol stress dynamic condition has become very common among humans over the past century and it's not going away, it's worldwide now as more and more humans join the rat race known as Western life style.

How does cortisol affect your low blood sugar? Cortisol tells the body to release stored energy from the muscles, joints, tendons and liver primarily. And why is cortisol released after your body starts running low on glucose? The stress hormone is released because of one evolutionary fact: the brain and nervous system cannot make or store glucose and glucose is the primary fuel of the brain. So cognition, the limbic system or emotional center of the brain, the cranial nerves affecting the senses—sight, hearing, smell, touch—innervation of the face, swallowing, speech, heart rate, breathing, stomach and bowels as well as peripheral nerves, all are profoundly vulnerable to low blood sugar states. This is true because the brain and nervous system cannot store or make glucose! When you start running low on fuel, the brain says: "Burn the furniture there's no fuel." Our body then goes into a stress response resulting in increased cortisol demand.

Depending upon the strength of your adrenals to produce cortisol as well as the vitality of your muscles and liver, you will either push through and not be affected greatly or feel wiped out by the later afternoon. What's more, cortisol demand increases with chronic blood sugar imbalance and elevated cortisol causes more insulin resistance. The survival hormone cortisol reduces the permeability of the body's cell membranes. This results in physiologic resistance to the intended effects of insulin. The pancreas must make more insulin to do the same work it previously did with less insulin. The body begins to develop insulin resistance. A high-circulating level of the anabolic hormone insulin tells the body, "Store for the future." Here is where insulin starts adding abdominal fat. The more abdominal fat we grow the more insulin we need to do the same amount of work because abdominal fat absorbs and stores insulin thus neutralizing its ability to regulate blood glucose levels. This negative feedback loop, created between high insulin-low blood sugar, low blood sugar-brain shock, brain shock-cortisol elevation and cortisol elevation and insulin resistance, leads to more insulin production and casts the body into a physiologic storm. More sugar, more insulin, more insulin, more fat, more fat more insulin, more insulin more fat. Also we have more sugar, more insulin, more insulin, more cortisol, more cortisol, more insulin resistance, more insulin resistance, and more insulin demand, more glucose swings. The physiologic storm grows and begins to erode vitality. Blood sugar instability can thus undermine the body's ability to heal. It's what I call being in a leaky boat amidst a storm at sea. The holes in the boat are the physical illnesses we endure, the injuries acute and chronic. The storm at sea is glycemic imbalance, situational stress or pain and inflammation, anything adding to cortisol demand. However, glycemic imbalance or blood sugar instability in particular is the most preventable. When it's added on top other stresses it can become and often is the last insult before capsizing.

In addition to whatever holes there are in the boat and the amount of energy and pharmaceutical buckets devoted to bailing out the boat, the physiologic storm at sea undermines our body's self-healing capabilities. All we do is bail harder and faster and get nowhere. There can be no enduring healing of chronic illness under these conditions. If the holes in the boat are medical problems or pre-disease states then much of what medicine provides us is a bigger, gold-plated bucket to bail with. When our body is in a physiologic storm, such as that created by chronic stresses, and then additionally it is subjected to hypoglycemia, it adds to an already high cortisol demand. The result is often that your body becomes so stressed that all you can do is bail out the boat—symptomatic treatments…

Harder!

Faster!

You don't have time to address the actual causes of your problems let along get your life back on course in directions you want to travel. You're just bailing out a leaky boat in a storm at sea, and the gold-plated bucket you're given is a pharmaceutical that keeps you afloat while all too often not addressing underlying causes.

Statistically, it's true that most arguments occur before dinner. Now you know why. Irritability, caused by glucose (sugar) imbalance, can trigger emotional reactions out of all proportion to what's before you. The main reason for mood, focus and irritability disturbances is the fact that the brain and entire nervous system cannot make or store glucose. A stress reaction occurs causing cortisol release that, among other things, causes the liver, muscles, tendons and other organs to release their stored energy because the brain's in trouble. Over thirty percent of humans are genetically predisposed to sugar/carbohydrate intolerance. Highly refined sugar intake is pushing the percentage of insulin resistance syndrome to nearly 60% of all Americans. The rest of the world isn't far behind. Obesity is everywhere. So is diabetes, so is heart disease, hypertension, cancers and numerous other chronic illnesses. It's not an accident, every system of your body is affected by this storm at sea.

Many times, there is a family history of diabetes, obesity, heart disease and stroke in people with carbohydrate intolerance. Even if you have no family history of diabetes, you can develop insulin resistance and hypo- or hyperglycemia after eating the wrong foods for years, for decades, as well as living a sedentary and/or stressed out life. When you have a family history of diabetes your pancreas tends to over-secrete insulin when you eat sugary foods. These are appropriately named "junk foods" because refined sugars are toxic anti-nutrients. Not only do refined carbs and sugars affect blood sugar but they also alter the bacterial flora which line our intestinal tracts, tens of trillions of benign bacteria, which aid digestion of nutrients from food and regulate the amount of inflammation and 70 percent of the adaptive immune function in your body.

Insulin lowers blood sugar, and high insulin level output can lower blood sugar very rapidly and very suddenly. What's worse is that in the long run, by the time you reach your thirties, forties and fifties and beyond, the insulin-producing beta cells of the pancreas can become overwhelmed and exhausted after secreting too much insulin for decades. The pancreas can then go from over-producing to under producing insulin. This condition is what is called type II or adult onset diabetes. This is a completely preventable disease.

But let's get back to the glucose or blood sugar roller coaster caused by eating high-glycemic, fast-releasing, "jet fuel" foods. Here's where the problems begin to multiply. When blood sugar drops rapidly in response to insulin secretion the brain reacts with a shock response. If you wanted to drive a hundred miles and you only put a dollar of gas in the tank your car would naturally just run out of fuel and stop dead. Why don't our bodies do this? The body keeps going because we have an emergency reserve, a system and adaptive capacity to store energy. The storage occurs especially in the liver, in the muscles and in the connective tissue. It is not stored in the brain and nervous system. Under stress conditions stored glucose is activated by cortisol from the adrenal glands and released into the blood stream to feed the brain and nervous system. There are other hormones involved with this balancing act, glucagon for example, but cortisol is your body's survival/stress hormone.

Then there's abdominal fat. Abdominal fat is not just fat. It is an endocrine organ interacting with the body's entire hormone system affecting not just insulin storage, demand and resistance but also producing leptins, inflammatory cytokines called adipokines (inflammatory cytokines produced in fat), and estrogens as well as storing toxins. In short, this is not good. Excess abdominal fat is associated with high blood pressure, diabetes, heart disease, cancer, arthritis, hormone imbalance, leaky small bowel, altered abdominal bacteria (microbiota) and eventually with chronic degenerative and autoimmune diseases or worse.

Over time, as you age, high cortisol demand, by stealing stored energy from our connective tissue and liver in order to give the brain needed fuel, can literally weaken your joints, making them creak and crack and become more prone to injury. The injuries are another form of stress and pain and so more cortisol is demanded. When I lived in New York City I treated many professional dancers. The ones who would not eat whole foods but rather drink fruit juice all day because they feared being replaced by an understudy if they gained weight were the ones who inevitably injured themselves more. Got hypoglycemia? Stretch and injure.

In this way the vicious cycle perpetuates itself along with more rapid aging. In fact, if you look back at the Holosystemic Mandala you'll be able to see how every system of your body is potentially vulnerable to being sabotaged by long-term high cortisol demand, aka stress in its various forms:

1.) Glycemic imbalance
2.) Injury, trauma shock, pain, infection, inflammation and allergic reactions
3.) Emotional, situational stress

How's your own personal Mandala doing?

The Epic Struggle
Insulin/Cortisol

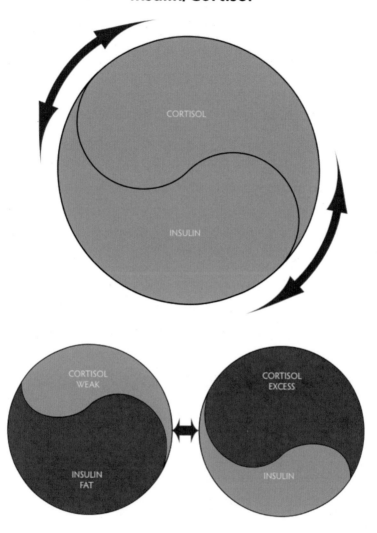

When either insulin or its agonist cortisol begin to overwhelm the capacity of the other to perform, you either drift into metabolic syndrome and later even diabetes or burn out your adrenals in a functional sense, or both. The outcome in terms of human misery and suffering, not to mention the loss of longevity and the cost to society of caring for preventable chronic illnesses is immense. It is made even more tragic since your body can heal these imbalances if you give them half a chance, if you eat fresh vegetables, fruits and lean proteins. Many of the problems considered normal signs of aging are preventable and reversible. By reducing stress, by eating and properly absorbing whole natural foods, through exercise, and, oh yes, laughter, we can reverse many symptoms we associate with "old age."

 Take Home Points

- The dynamic relationship between insulin and glucose blood sugar levels is of critical importance in both the cause and prevention of disease.

- Maintaining proper glycemic control creates a fundamental solid foundation for enabling your body's self-healing potential.

- Over time high cortisol demand diminishes the adrenal glands' capacity and vitality begins to wane.

- Cortisol is released after your body starts running low on glucose.

- Cortisol demand increases with chronic blood sugar imbalance and elevated cortisol causes more insulin resistance, leading to abdominal fat.

- Prevent a glucose or blood sugar roller coaster by avoiding high-glycemic, fast-releasing, "jet fuel" foods. However, as you will see with Laurence's case study below, simply avoiding low-glycemic foods isn't always the answer.

Your Self-Healing Body in Action

Case Study #2:
A Mistaken Diagnosis of Diabetes, Stroke, and Congestive Heart Failure

Three months before 53-year-old Laurence, as I will call him, first arrived in my office he had visited the emergency room with symptoms of a stroke. He had had a severe headache, right upper and lower extremity numbness and weakness, numbness in the jaw, right facial weakness, and slurring of speech. After a number of hours in the ER, they diagnosed him with a hypertensive crisis, a transient ischemic attack (TIA or mini stroke), and cerebral vasospasm (spasm in the artery of the brain).

Laurence weighed about 290 pounds and he was 5'9". A coagulation test revealed his coagulation time was rapid, which means his blood was thick. His blood sugar was very high—391—so they diagnosed him with new onset diabetes mellitus type 2. His sodium was low, his potassium was low, his chloride was low. This made

WHAT HAPPENS DURING A TIA?

During a TIA or mini stroke, blood flow is temporarily blocked from reaching the brain by either an atherosclerotic plaque or a blood clot that has migrated from the heart. Usually if you throw a clot—in other words, the clot moves away from your heart—you're going to block a small artery in the brain. And because the blood can't flow, the whole artery goes into spasm. That creates a headache. The blocked artery also causes the part of the brain that operates the motor cortex to be deprived of its blood supply and oxygen, affecting the ability to move and causing numbness. In Laurence's case, the TIA affected the left side of his brain, which caused the right side of the body to feel numb.

sense since what happens with diabetes is that you urinate a lot because you're throwing off glucose, ketones, and acids. This pulls out electrolytes and dehydrates you severely. So, Laurence was depleted.

His hemoglobin A1c (HbA1c) was high at 10.5. Normal is less than 5.7. HbA1C is a way to measure blood sugar over time, so based on his elevated HbA1c Laurence's average blood sugar over the previous three months would have been well over 200. Typical of diabetes and insulin resistance, his triglycerides (circulating fats) were high at 332. His cholesterol tested at 227, which, in my mind wasn't all that bad, but the emergency room physicians diagnosed him with high cholesterol.

> ## WHAT ARE KETONES?
>
> *Ketones are produced when the body uses fat as an energy source rather than carbohydrates. They're produced when a person is eating a low-carbohydrate diet or when the body is unable to use glucose effectively.*

By the time Laurence left the ER, most of his primary symptoms had resolved. The ER physician diagnosed him with new onset diabetes mellitus type 2, obesity, high cholesterol, TIAs and hypertensive coronary artery disease. They also believed he had congestive heart failure and decreased ventricular function; in other words, the heart was weak and couldn't pump effectively. He was given a number of drugs—blood pressure and blood sugar lowering meds and a statin drug—and was told to go home.

Soon after his trip to the ER, Laurence sought the help of an anthroposophical medical doctor, a type of physician who evaluates not only the physical body but also the psyche and personality of the patient. Unfortunately, that doctor put him on a diet of raw cow's milk, a lot of grains, and very little animal protein. Laurence's blood sugar continued to climb. He was starting to get palpitations. He had shortness of breath and low energy.

Three months after his stroke, he came to see me, and I spent two hours learning about his situation, as I do with all my new patients. I asked myself why was he so sick when he was eating all these good natural products—fresh-from-the-farm eggs, fresh milk and whole grains? He wasn't eating high-glycemic, refined carbohydrates. Based on what I was about to find out about his health, I later realized eating high-glycemic, refined foods probably would have killed him.

> ## THE GLYCEMIC INDEX
>
> *The glycemic index (GI) refers to how much a given food raises blood sugar and insulin levels. The higher the GI, the more insulin is demanded. For instance, white flour has a glycemic index of 90, glucose has a GI of 100. Whole wheat has a GI of 60.*

What Was Wrong with Laurence?

Laurence came to me because he was eating all this good food and not only was he not losing weight—he was still sick. Why? That's a good question. And I did a couple of things in order to find out. I gave him the same glycemic questionnaire you'll find in this book. His glycemic questionnaire didn't reveal a lot of symptoms I would have expected to see in someone with blood sugar and insulin as high as his was. The questionnaire revealed he had shortness of breath, frequent urination, high blood pressure, cold hands and feet, and dizziness. He was avoiding refined carbohydrates (sugars) so that a lot of his symptoms were reduced. However, his blood sugar was through the roof, his blood pressure was still high, and he was starting to get palpitations and heart symptoms again. He had allergies and wheezed a lot.

Based upon what he was telling me, I ordered some testing. His gluten IgG, which is a chronic antibody to gluten, should have been less than 2. It was elevated at 4.2. This indicated he had acquired gluten sensitivity.

Another test revealed his fasting blood sugar was 218 but his insulin was 41. What does that mean? Diabetes? I don't think so. He had too much insulin. With a glucose of 218 his ideal insulin would be 21.8 or less. It was 41, almost twice that. He had way too much insulin. And he had elevated blood sugar. This condition is not strictly speaking diabetes. It is called metabolic syndrome and has risk factors for heart disease, including an excessive amount of abdominal fat, high triglycerides, blood sugar, and blood pressure, and low levels of the "good" cholesterol HDL.

Both elevated insulin and elevated glucose can cause elevated triglycerides. Most work ups for patients with Laurence's symptoms look at blood sugar but not insulin levels. When

DIFFERENCE BETWEEN CELIAC DISEASE AND ACQUIRED GLUTEN SENSITIVITY

Acquired gluten sensitivity describes people who experience celiac-like symptoms but who don't have the same antibodies to gluten nor the intestinal damage that occurs in celiac disease. Acquired gluten sensitivity is considered to be an innate immune response rather than an autoimmune adaptive immune response. An estimated 18 million Americans suffer from gluten sensitivity—six times the number who have celiac disease. Celiac is a needle in a haystack. Acquired gluten sensitivity is the haystack.

an adult presents with a blood sugar of 300 and the HA1c is high, doctors will most likely diagnose diabetes type II or "adult onset diabetes." This is the most common type of diabetes and it is usually completely preventable with the correct diet, nutrients and lifestyle adjustments. In Laurence's case, as with many in his situation it is essential to look at insulin and glucose ratios. The ideal ratio between glucose and insulin would be around 10 to 1. For a person whose blood sugar is 300, at most the insulin level should be 30. If blood sugar was 100, the ideal insulin would be between ten and four. Less insulin than four would suggest insulin insufficiency. If the insulin level is 200 and the blood sugar is 300 how could it be diabetes? By definition, diabetes is insulin insufficiency as well as elevated blood sugar. Laurence had too much insulin, and to give him insulin as a treatment would have drastically exacerbated his condition.

If you don't look at the insulin side of the equation, and diagnose diabetes based on high blood sugar levels only then prescribe insulin injections, the patient will be condemned to a cycle of more and more insulin which grows more fat which absorbs the insulin which keeps upping the need for more insulin—a true negative feedback loop—and irreversible insulin-resistant diabetes. Laurence's case is a classic illustration of insulin resistance, metabolic syndrome, and reaching a state of borderline diabetes. We were able to pull Laurence back from the edge by understanding that he had too much insulin and not too little. So how did we use this information to help Laurence's body heal? I'll explain in a minute.

A Slam Dunk in Blood Sugar

Laurence's high insulin and blood sugar levels and his gluten sensitivity pointed to the fact he was an example of someone with carbohydrate intolerance, which I first learned about when I worked with Dr. Atkins in the early '80s. In those days we didn't know all the facts about insulin resistance and its system wide effects on the body.

Carbohydrate intolerance is basically just another way to describe insulin resistance. People who have carb intolerance and a family history of diabetes often tend to overexpress insulin in response to carbohydrates especially sugar-saturated refined carbs such as white rice and white flour. When the pancreas over-reacts with too much insulin the effect can be a roller coaster ride of too high then too low blood glucose levels, a slam dunk of their blood sugar. Their blood sugar goes way up, their insulin goes way up, their blood sugar doesn't respond, the insulin goes up higher, and finally the blood sugar crashes while their insulin is still way high. This causes brain and nervous system shock leading to a multitude of possible mental, emotional and physiologic symptoms.

These symptoms, including feeling faint, extreme lethargy and fatigue, tingling and disruption of nerves, heart palpitations, sweats, poor concentration, irritability and shock are all symptoms familiar to people with insulin dependent diabetes who have overdosed on insulin—a medical emergency. Since the brain and nervous system cannot make or store glucose they are both vulnerable to low-glucose conditions. The brain says "burn the furniture there's no fuel" and the survival hormone cortisol is secreted from the adrenals. Cortisol raises blood sugar, among other effects, by taking stored energy from the liver, muscles, tendons, joints and organs. Stress reactions like this increase cortisol demand over time and can deplete energy reserves and healing vitality. The survival hormone cortisol tells the body to release stored energy for a glucose-starved brain. This is our evolved reserve energy system when we lack fuel—shock and awe leading to lack and stall.

If hypoglycemia occurs regularly due to poor diet, excess insulin and other stresses, there can be a gradual erosion of adrenal vitality so that crashes become more severe. Moreover, it is an established scientific fact that cortisol increases insulin resistance. In Laurence's case this situation caused symptoms of stroke, heart attack, peripheral neuropathy, brain fog, poor memory and emotional volatility—the slam dunk in blood sugar.

Eating high-glycemic foods causes insulin resistance over time. But Laurence was eating the *low*-glycemic variety of carbohydrates. In his case his pancreas was getting overwhelmed. Laurence couldn't deal with *any* type of carb—high or low glycemic. And yet he was eating a high-carb, low-protein diet, the opposite of what he needed. Not only did this push his endocrine hormone insulin secretion to excess, it also diminished the exocrine digestive enzyme function of the pancreas to deficiency. Laurence had developed severe abdominal bloating, gas and irritable bowel symptoms with his diet.

A Physiologic Snowstorm

A key player in Laurence's inability to deal with carbs was his obesity. Abdominal fat absorbs insulin and neutralizes it so the pancreas has to work harder in order to put out more insulin. The insulin isn't getting to where it needs to go, which is at cellular insulin receptors so cells can take the glucose out of the blood stream. Abdominal fat is a sponge absorbing insulin, not letting it do what it has to do, and therefore putting more and more stress on the pancreas. That's why if Laurence had continued to eat even low-glycemic carbs he would have fried his insulin-producing beta pancreatic cells. This would surely have become real diabetes.

Insulin is an anabolic hormone that tells the body to store for the future, because it might be a long winter, and there might not be enough food. As noted above, abdominal fat absorbs insulin and insulin stimulates abdominal fat production. This negative feedback loop leads to elevated insulin whether or not you've eaten anything. Your pancreas is gunning its engine at the stop light in neutral. Thus, insulin levels remain elevated with insulin resistance. This is why metabolic syndrome or insulin resistance can eventually lead to diabetes. The insulin-producing beta cells of the pancreas can become exhausted. After a number of years diabetes can result. Alternately, many in this fix just put on weight, develop chronic degenerative diseases and negatively impact both the quality and quantity of their life.

Abdominal fat is a key element. Eat refined sugars such as corn-syrup-sweetened drinks, fruit juices, refined grains stripped of nutrients, essential fatty acids and fiber and the result is insulin overproduction and increasing abdominal fat. The effect on blood sugar can be drastic because there is a disconnect between blood sugar and insulin. Normally as blood sugar goes up insulin goes up, and when blood sugar goes down insulin immediately drops. However, with metabolic syndrome, blood sugar goes up, insulin goes up, blood sugar doesn't go down so insulin goes up more until a delayed response to much higher levels of insulin cause a sudden and often severe crash in blood sugar. This creates a cortisol stress response leading to many symptom presentations that would lead a doctor down a pathway of diagnosing a wide array of other pathologies. Making an accurate diagnosis becomes like trying to find a tennis ball in a physiologic snowstorm. To accurately read the terrain we first need to calm the physiologic turbulence. What we're left with may be pathology of some kind, but in a glycemic-insulin storm it's hard to accurately read anything.

A Primary Culprit Behind Laurence's Problems

Laurence also had a history of gastric distress, including heartburn and gastritis. This, along with the carbohydrate intolerance, pointed to a leaky gut as the cause of many of his problems. There is a very strong connection between carbohydrate intolerance, leaky small bowel and small bowel intestinal overgrowth (SIBO) or small bowel bacterial overgrowth. The connection is based upon the science of the microbiota of the human GI system. Our bodies are made up of about ten trillion human cells, but we have 100 trillion bacteria on the surface of our skin and in our gut. We're ten times more bacteria than we are human cells. The barrier between the outside world passing through us in the bowel and the inner world of the blood stream is created by connective tissue that seals the cellular intestinal lining.

Those normal bacteria and that barrier—known as the microbiome and normal cellular integrity—are an interface between the outside world and the inside world of our skin, gut, respiratory and urinary tracts. The interface between bacteria and the mucosal lining of the gut is inseparable. One defines the other in a reciprocal way. The bacteria define us and we define the bacteria. In fact, 70 percent or more of our adaptive immune system is based upon that interaction.

If the ecosystem of the gut like the soil in the garden is rich and well composted and full of nutrients then what grows there will be beneficial. But if the ecosystem (meaning the mucosal lining of the gut) is inflamed due to antibiotics, gastritis, fundamental or acquired gluten sensitivity, allergic reaction or insults like parasites or yeast overgrowth, too many sugars, too many antibiotics, and various other insults to our system there is a breakdown in the connective tissue, a loss of integrity and filtering ability with the result that partially digested foods leak into the blood stream. This can provoke inflammatory immune and autoimmune reactions every time we eat. Over time this condition not only damages the immune function of the intestinal lining, it also changes the types of bacteria which grow in the gut leading to even more damage and malabsorption. Under these conditions the more we eat of any one type of food the more likely we are to develop a reaction to it. The inflammation in the mucosal lining erodes the barrier between outside and inside worlds and helps damage the immune function of those cells. This is because in the digestive system immune function and structure are one and the same. The structure of the immune cells in the gut creates a barrier between the outside world within the gut and the inside world in the blood stream, necessary for proper digestion. It's the soil bed that the bacteria inhabit and interact with and that the food comes through in a filtered way to emerge into the blood stream as a recognizable nutrient for the body to use.

Carbohydrate, sugar intolerance can both cause and be the cause of malabsorption, sensitivity to foods and leaky gut. This is one of the leading factors involved in autoimmune diseases such as celiac, colitis, irritable bowel, Crohn's, as well as Hashimoto's thyroiditis, arthritis, psoriasis, eczema and migraines. Partially digested foods in the blood stream caused by leaky small intestine form immune complexes. These immune complexes can cause further damage to bowel wall and activate and perpetuate bowel disorders. The immune complexes can also travel through the Portal venous system through the liver then circulate throughout the body and deposit in different organs and tissues. The immune system attacks that deposited inflammatory toxic immune complex leading to arthritis in the joints, psoriasis or eczema when deposited in the skin, Hashimoto's thyroiditis when deposited in the thyroid, etc., etc.

As with all things in nature, when you look at a cloud and can ask, "What caused that cloud?" there are as many partially correct answers as there are many causes. Few things in nature have that satisfying linear cause effect we humans crave in trying to explain what is before us. There are complex systems from which things are emerging. One can look at the cloud and say it looks like rain, or looks like it might be a thunderstorm, but you don't know exactly when or where the storm is going to emerge. And that unpredictability is biology—it's messy, it's wobbly, it's a cloud.

Based on this unpredictability it's impossible to say where an autoimmune disease will show up. You can't say if you eat this wheat it's going to go right to your thyroid. If you have a family history of thyroiditis or if you have a family history of autoimmune disease or of diabetes then it's much more likely you can predict accurately, but a lot of people never develop autoimmune disease. And a lot of our ability to quell inflammatory response and to heal has to do with our own inherited genetic expression.

Healing is not just about what it is and where it is located in the body, it's also about having the vitality to mount an adequate healing response. And Laurence didn't have that vitality. What he

WHAT ARE SECRETORY IgAs?

Secretory IgAs are immune antibodies created by the mucosal lining of the gut. These antibodies help protect us from infection.

did have was a bad case of leaky gut. He could eat one grain and the next week eat another grain and whatever he ate the most of he reacted to. It reached the point he was fermenting and reacting to almost everything he ate.

We established that Laurence had leaky gut in part by ordering a SED rate test to detect inflammation. The SED rate should be less than 20. His SED rate was high at 55, indicating he had inflammation. We also tested for *Helicobacter Pylori*, a normal bacterium in the stomach, but when conditions allow and *H. Pylori* overgrows ulcers and gastritis can emerge. In a comprehensive stool and saliva test Laurence's secretory IgA levels were suppressed.

However, his *H. Pylori* antibody levels were not elevated in spite of a clear history of gastritis. The secretory IgA should have been 40 to 880. They were low at 10. That told me his gut immune system had deteriorated. A person who has autoimmune disease will often have an elevated secretory IgA. Laurence, however, had a suppression of immune function probably due to chronic inflammation and immune exhaustion. A warning to us to treat the person and pay attention to their history and symptoms rather than just treat lab results.

A Brewery in His Gut

In the comprehensive stool analysis results we were able to pinpoint an important cause and effect of Laurence's leaky gut. The stool analysis revealed a large overgrowth of yeast in his intestines. He had high levels of four species of candida. He was a fermentation factory. The carbohydrates Laurence ate, whether low- or high-glycemic, refined or unrefined all fermented in the presence of excess yeast. His gut was a brewery. And why was he growing so much yeast? Because he was sweet. His blood sugar was high. Yeasts love sugar. So even though he wasn't eating a lot of sugar he was yeasty.

There was an ecological imbalance in the microflora of his bowel. The fermentation process was irritating his gut and the irritation in the gut was perpetuating leaky bowel and the leaky bowel caused more reactivity and the reactivity caused more inflammation and the inflammation led to more abnormal species growing in the bowel—a negative feedback loop to be sure. Negative feedback loops are the real key. If you can steadily and gradually shut down that negative feedback loop the body will heal. Like a car tire stuck in the snow, if you get a little traction the car will move out of a rut. In the same way, the body can and will heal. The blockage, the impasse, the negative feedback loop of inflammation and the amplification of this inflammation by abnormal bacteria all combine to perpetuate ill health.

Emerging Heart Trouble

Laurence's BNP (brain natriuretic peptide), which is used to help diagnose and monitor congestive heart failure, was just slightly elevated. Normal is less than 100, Laurence's value was 130. When someone is in the middle of congestive heart failure

(CHF) they have a BNP of 300 or more. Someone who has chronic CHF will probably hover around 200. Laurence's BNP of 130 indicated there was some stress on the heart, but not full- blown CHF.

WHAT IS BNP?

BNP is a brain-generated diuretic that tries to get rid of fluid when the brain senses the heart is in trouble.

There were, however, other indications that Laurence's heart was affected by his high blood sugar and insulin resistance. His C-reactive protein, which is a marker of cardiovascular risk and inflammation, should be less than 3. His was 30. And his homocysteine, an amino acid that is linked to cardiovascular risk, was 19 when it ideally should be around 8. These lab results often occur with diabetes. With elevated blood glucose the blood becomes thickened and sticky. Arteries and tissues grow irritated, glucose starts sticking to the cells, gumming up membranes which signals more cycles of inflammation and immune attack. This inflammatory process disrupts methylation in the liver. Methylation is a process that recycles the toxic free radical homocysteine into SAMe. SAMe is an energy-rich molecule like little battery packs that assist in the production of energy throughout the body by helping produce the universal energy molecule ATP. Methylation is important in detoxification, brain biochemistry and genetic expression. When methylation is disrupted, homocysteine piles up on the deck, increasing the risk of heart disease along with other health problems.

How Laurence's Body Started to Heal Itself

To summarize, we learned that Laurence had an incredible amount of inflammation, poor methylation (and consequently impaired detox capacity and energy production capacity), elevated glucose and insulin resistance, leaky small bowel with yeast overgrowth and allergies to gluten and many other foods. We put Laurence on a rotational diet of lean proteins, vegetables, and some berries with almost no carbohydrates. He drank a lot of water with a little lemon in it to alkalinize and to prevent dehydration on the ketogenic diet he was following. He was allowed to have some small portions of non-glutinous grains such as quinoa and brown rice. The primary objective of this diet wasn't to help Laurence drop weight quickly though this surely took place. The primary objective was to stabilize his glucose, re-sensitize his body to insulin and reduce cortisol demand and stress. Incidentally this diet did help shed inches and pounds. The more fat Laurence burned off the more efficiently his insulin controlled blood sugar levels. His blood pressure came down, his sleep improved, his energy improved and his blood sugars normalized. Most importantly, Laurence felt like a new man.

We also started Laurence on 200 mcg of chromium pico-linate and 100 mg alpha lipoic acid with each meal. These nutrients help re-sensitization to insulin. We also gave him a few formulas to help reduce blood sugar. Laurence's vitamin D level was extremely low, so we started him on 5,000 i.u. daily of vitamin D3. Vitamin D3 is an important hormone-like vitamin needed for immune function, diabetes prevention, regulation against autoimmune diseases, as well as bone health. Laurence took low-dose probiotics including a benign yeast *Saccharomyces Boulardii*, pancreatic digestive enzymes with betaine hydrochloride, omega-3 from flax, GLA (primrose oil), vitamin D3/K2 along with the amino acid l-glutamine, aloe vera and herbs that soothe inflammation and heal up the holes in the gut. Because he had tested high for an inflamma-tory protein involved in injury repair known as fibrinogen, we started Laurence on nattokinase, an anti-inflammatory enzyme that reduces fibrinogen and reduces stickiness in the blood. That was phase I which lasted several weeks. During phase II we continued as in phase I but started to reduce Laurence's yeast overgrowth, we started Laurence on some anti-candida herbs along with psyllium bentonite colon cleanser to keep things moving, to scrub the bowel and osmotically pull out mucous and toxins and organisms that don't belong in the gut. In addition, Laurence started taking high doses of multiple probiotic bacteria to encourage new healthy bowel integrity and function.

By doing this, we helped heal the soil beds of his intestines by implanting beneficial bacteria in addition to eliminating abnormal species like candida. Bombing bugs alone will not reverse inflammation and promote healing. Killing abnormal bacteria is all too often the linear approach taken by "standard of care" medical models—identify a bug and bomb it. We cannot take a swamp, spray DDT all over it and expect the mosquitoes to stay away forever. They're going to come back and the ones that come back are going to be DDT resistant because the ecosystem hasn't changed. Instead, we need to drain the swamp, improve the soil and create conditions for benign organisms to grow and for the proper digestion to take place. Through diet, probiotics, and nutrients to heal gut inflammation and repair the integrity of the gut ecosystem, a more comprehensive and sustainable approach to healing emerges.

Once Laurence became less weak and stabilized he did a flush to cleanse the liver. This helped him eliminate toxins from his liver and gallbladder and also improved his energy and digestion of fats.

Laurence's Dramatic Response

By November, eight weeks into his recovery, Laurence's response to treatment was noteworthy. His energy improved dramatically within a week. His glucose was consistently less than 120 upon arising in the morning. He dropped down to 230 pounds, a loss of roughly 60 pounds over a couple of months. His blood sugar correspondingly started behaving normally because he didn't have so much abdominal fat and he wasn't provoking his pancreas with all the carbs. His irritable bowel symptoms had vanished as well. Basically, his body was telling him this was the right thing to do, the right direction to take for healing. Laurence didn't have symptoms of heart problems. His wheezing had stopped, his allergies had stopped, his headaches had stopped, his numbness had stopped, his neurological symptoms had gone away, his blood pressure had normalized, he did not have diabetes, and he was not on any medications.

At that point he was a different person. He started working again. His wife had been doing everything for six to seven months. She was exhausted. Laurence was so happy that a giant smile lit up his face. And that made my day. It was so pleasing to be able to reach into that maelstrom and grab a handle. I didn't really do that much, just a few modifications and a few targeted nutrients and the downward disease cycles flipped to upward healing and repair cycles. Laurence's body engaged its own self-healing capacity.

Often the good physician acts as a midwife in the healing process. We can help cure, yet nature's self-organizing energy is what heals. I have observed this turn around hundreds of times over thirty-six years of clinical practice. People present like balls of knotted strings, their various symptoms complexes all knotted together. Interestingly, if we pick out one or two essential causative elements and gently pull on those strings the whole ball of symptoms begins to unravel. Biology and nature are holographic, interdependent clouds. Everything is interconnected, the whole contains and is contained in the part. If we heal our gut we reduce the antigenic challenges of foods, we reduce inflammation, we regain a good digestive ecosystem, we improve our immune system, we start losing weight, blood pressure comes down, blood sugar stabilizes, insulin demand shrinks and instead of falling into disease-causing downward spirals we set our body towards upward-healing cycles. In other words, we empower our body to engage its self-healing capacity. And that's the essence of your self-healing body.

CHAPTER 6

A Special Dynamic—Cortisol/Thyroid Function

The very interactive nature of your biological systems demands that you pay attention to them. This self-acknowledgement allows you to remain centered while you move through life with gifts to share with others. Pausing to take a deep breath allows a resetting of the adrenal stress response. It alters both cortisol demand as well as your conscious presence and calm. Take a deep breath. While you cannot change many things, including the emotional biochemistry of your mother or your father during your early life in utero, while you cannot alter your past traumas, your shock upon entering this life or leaving it, the simple act of knowing, of acknowledging these traumas while taking a deep breath will reset your survival brain and allow your intelligence, calm, compassion and wisdom to emerge. If you breathe in the moment then you will reset your internal thermostats, your thyroid and your adrenals, to a more comfortable temperature. It's at this moment that your adrenals relax and reset. It is here that your adrenals can begin to heal, with a deep and slow, healing breath.

At this point I want to mention the dynamic relationship between cortisol and thyroid function. Rather than seeing the adrenal glands and thyroid as separate organs, the holosystemic, fractal and holographic nature of your biology demand that you also appreciate the interactive nature of these two catabolic or energy-accelerating and energy-spending organs. The very interactive nature of your biological systems demand that you acknowledge the dynamic relationship between adrenals and thyroid systems: the cortisol production, regulation and uptake and the thyroid production, regulation and cellular level uptake.

As cortisol demand rises chronically over time it begins to negatively affect the uptake of thyroid hormone at the cellular level everywhere in your body. There can be no separation of thyroid from adrenals and adrenals from thyroid. Just as cortisol can contribute to insulin resistance so elevated cortisol (i.e. stress) can block the uptake of thyroid thus placing increased demands on the thyroid to produce greater amounts of thyroid hormone. This chronic stress condition, be it psycho-social stress, pain, inflammation, trauma, allergy or blood sugar imbalance can affect both adrenal and thyroid functions individually and all together at all levels. Even as blood, saliva and urine levels of the two hormones remain within normal limits, the physiologic responses become muted or deficient due to the close catabolic nature and interaction between the adrenals and the thyroid. Whether you are predisposed by genetics or because of your diet, chronic gut inflammation or an autoimmune inflammation, whether the thyroid is stronger or whether the adrenals are stronger, the weakest organ will drain the other in real physiologic and perhaps even pathologic ways.

Preventable!

It is rarely a case of either/or and most often a case of which organs are affected. In medicine as in all of science and life, if we don't look, we won't see, and the way we look, the types of tests we use, their sensitivity as well as their intent will determine what we can finally understand. A problem with modern medicine's approach to understanding physiologic phenomena is that most standard medical testing is oriented towards pathology. This is a good thing and yet this is also a very limiting and limited view of reality. How often has the patient complained of multiple symptoms, the doctor obligingly draws blood and urine for testing but the results all return 100% normal, yet "normal" is not the same as "optimal." The physician, trained to diagnose disease, then says, "I can find nothing wrong with you." What that means is that, "By our pathology-oriented standards of assessing your condition and limited models for integrating the body's complex systems we can find no observable disease state requiring medical intervention."

In fact, all of Western medicine is oriented towards determining pathology. Thetests are standardized to focus above the water line. It's like looking only at the part of the iceberg that's visible. What is visible has already become a "problem," meaning a pre-disease state or an overt disease. Chronic illness is often at the waterline. Sometimes it is overtly diagnosable and then again often the classically described prodrome or syndrome never emerges fully. This is because the symptoms are a warning telling us that the body can no longer regulate itself properly. (This is red on the mandala.)

Put in another way, when you take a medicine to suppress symptoms you are ignoring warning signs saying, "Go Slow

Dangerous Icebergs Ahead." When you take medications to suppress symptoms then go back to party on the deck you are at risk of developing even worse problems. You are at risk of sinking the ship. Is it any surprise that something worse often emerges from this limited strategy? How could that have happened?" It's a surprise only because you didn't bother to read the signs.

Normal testing often misses these borderline, chronic cases (orange on the mandala) because of the way we look at and for problems. Our perspective frames and also limits understanding of biology. We see the part of the iceberg in sight. The greater portion of the total iceberg, the part that is below the water, the conditions leading toward and away from disease are often not on the physician's radar. Western medical models often lack structures that would allow or encourage complex system analysis. Intellectual questioning modeled not only upon isolation and definition of distinctness of pathologies, but also upon interactivity of body systems, optimal versus normal and vital versus depleted are sorely needed. One can have all "normal" test results but "optimal" test results are something quite different. To diagnose illness is one thing but to prevent illness is quite another thing again. Complex systems and emergent dynamics actually exist in life. Our diagnostic capacity is very much limited by our mental modeling. What you look for you may find. If you don't bother to look to begin with, then you are bound to have limited insight. If you do not appreciate the self-organizing energy of your body you turn real biology into mechanics. *The good physician can cure, the excellent physician can prevent illness but only nature can heal.*

In traditional Western diagnosis we have become so specialized that the tongue is not related to the stomach, the stomach not related to the bowel, the bowel not related to the joints or other diseases emerging from the chronic inflammatory conditions. This not only defies simple common sense, this view also defies the holographic nature of the universe we are a part of. How could it be other than all inter-related? One just has to look closely and with keener sensitivity to see the patterns of inter-connectedness emerging everywhere. This self-organizational energy has spiral, mathematical symmetry and is the reason the second Law of Thermodynamics, the law of entropy or energy loss doesn't begin to explain where the self-organizing energy came from to begin with. You cannot have entropy unless you first have self-organizing energy and matter. These dynamics play out in our daily lives.

 Take Home Points

- Pausing to take a deep breath allows a resetting of the adrenal stress response, allowing your adrenals to relax and reset. It alters both cortisol demand as well as your conscious presence and calm.

- There can be no separation of thyroid from adrenals and adrenals from thyroid. Just as cortisol can contribute to insulin resistance so elevated cortisol (i.e. stress) can block the uptake of thyroid thus placing increased demands on the thyroid to produce greater amounts of thyroid hormone.

- Chronic stress, be it psycho-social stress, pain, inflammation, trauma, allergy or blood sugar imbalance, can affect both adrenal and thyroid functions individually and all together at all levels.

- In traditional Western diagnosis we have become so specialized that the tongue is not related to the stomach, the stomach not related to the bowel, the bowel not related to the joints or other diseases emerging from the chronic inflammatory conditions. This not only defies simple common sense, this view also defies the holographic nature of the universe we are a part of.

CHAPTER 7

What's Happening in Your Own Body?

I'd like to ask you to take a few moments to look over a *Glycemic Questionnaire* that I use with all my patients. Try filling it out in order to get a feel for how balanced or unbalanced your blood sugar may be. Go ahead, take a look, and then check the level of intensity of each symptom in the list:

0= Never

1= Occasional

2= Frequently with more intensity

3= All the time and very intensely.

Go ahead, I'll wait for you.

Name_____ Date_____

A Few Questions About How You Feel

Check off each one of the symptoms in one of the columns to indicate the degree of severity which best applies to you. A check in column **0 = NONE, 1 = MILD, 2 = MODERATE, 3 = SEVERE.** Please use the designated space on the bottom of the page if you have any other problems not listed or if you choose to expand on your answer.

0	1	2	3		0	1	2	3	
				Abnormal craving for sweets					Heart palpitations (fast beats)
				Afternoon headaches					Heart pain
				Allergies					Highly emotional
				Awaken after a few hrs. sleep and can't return easily					"Pin and Needle" sensation (where_____)
				Aware of breathing heavily					Insomnia
				Bad Dreams					Joint pain (where_____)
				Backache					Lack of energy
				Blurred Vision					Leg pain when walking
				Brown spots/Bronzing of skin					Leg pain when resting
				Bruise easily					Low or High Blood Pressure
				Can't decide easily					Indigestion
				Can't get started in morning					Poor memory/ability to concentrate
				Chills					Phlebitis
				Chronic Fatigue					Pain when rotating neck or hips
				Colds hand and feet					Reduced initiative
				Chest pain (where _____)					Ringing in ears
				Chronic nervous exhaustion					Sleepy after meals
				Decreased vision/clarity					Sleepy during the day
				Decreased hearing					Shortness of breath
				Decreased sex drive					Swelling in ankles
				Dizziness or light headedness					Swishing sounds in ears
				Dry skin					Tired too often
				Dry hair					Urinary problems, (please explain_____)
				Dry or brittle nails					Varicose veins
				Earaches					Weakness
				Fatigue					Worry or feel insecure
				Forgetful					Hand(s) tremble
				Get "shaky" if hungry					Head pain

Use space below to add or describe any complaints or problems you may have.

_____

_____

_____

Now that you have reviewed the questionnaire it may feel a bit more personal when I tell you the other implications of the cortisol/insulin dynamics. Just to summarize what we've been covering:

The more insulin you make the more abdominal fat you grow and abdominal fat is not simply fat. Abdominal fat is an endocrine organ. It not only stores insulin and renders it ineffective thus making your pancreas work ever harder, but this fat also produces substances called cytokines that are inflammatory, cardiovascular damaging, joint injuring and immune system disrupting. Additionally, this insulin stimulated abdominal fat produces glucose-generating leptins that can make the liver raise blood sugar levels in response to inflammatory stress. Abdominal fat also stores carcinogenic, free radical forms of estrogen and many other pro-inflammatory adipokines or fat-based inflammatory factors. All of these—cytokines, leptins, estrones and adipokines—pre-seed and lead to all sorts of chronic degenerative diseases including cancer.

Insulin is as much to blame for the bad side effects associated with diabetes as are elevated sugar levels. In the case of the alarmingly common metabolic syndrome, where diet causes overproduction of insulin, as well as in diabetics who inject insulin, insulin resistance can and does occur. Insulin resistance can happen in anyone due to overconsumption of refined carbohydrates and sugars. Insulin and abdominal fat are at the core of many medical problems. The increasing demand for more insulin caused by insulin-generating, high-glycemic value foods causes increased abdominal fat accumulation around the waist. It's a commonly observable syndrome, now even reaching into populations usually not affected such as professional athletes.

Since abdominal fat neutralizes the effectiveness of insulin, insulin resistance results. This becomes the metabolic equivalent of the beta cells of the pancreas gunning their engines in neutral at a stop light day and night. When I measure insulin levels in these patients they invariably have glucose/insulin levels far above an optimal ratio of around 10 to one. When I measure my patients' fasting glucose and it's 100 for example, and the insulin is 20, normal but far from optimal, this means there is a good probability that the person is on the road to insulin resistance. Insulin/glucose levels and the symptoms a person experiences tell the full story.

When necessary, I ask my patients to do a 5-hour glucose tolerance test with serial insulin levels included. I believe it is far more instructive and medically valuable to track serial insulin levels at the same time glucose levels are taken. This test, if indicated, can tell you a lot about your glycemic control, your ability to metabolize sugars and carbohydrates as well as forewarn you about insulin resistance or even borderline diabetes. Hemoglobin A1C can give you an average blood sugar level over the past three months, the glucose/insulin tolerance test can dramatically chart insulin resistance and pre-diabetic glycemic/insulin imbalances. It can demonstrate how persons with somewhat elevated glucose levels are not under-producing but rather over-producing insulin. I have numerous patients already diagnosed with diabetes and who were told they needed insulin injection therapy experience a complete reversal of this condition after testing demonstrated that they, in fact, had too much insulin, but their body was in insulin resistance so the blood sugars were running high.

The Glucose Tolerance Test involves measuring fasting glucose and insulin levels then administering 44 grams or more of a glucose drink or high-glycemic meal. Following this I take blood glucose and insulin levels at the ½ hour mark, then hourly for up to 5 hours. The patient's subjective signs and symptoms are observed and recorded by the attending nurse as well as by the patient. I do not recommend nor need to perform this test on weaker patients since it is rigorous and can cause depleted patients a significant setback. The results of this test, however, can yield a tremendous amount of insight into a person's dominant metabolic functions as well as expose an important cause of multiple symptom complexes. Often random glucose/insulin levels appear normal in patients with multiple glycemic/insulin imbalance symptoms. The glucose tolerance/serial insulin test can be a definitive diagnostic tool and change lives.

The chart on the next page is an example of the graphic information obtainable from this test. Plotting out these curves and explaining the relationships between glucose levels and insulin levels can provide a person with a valuable wake up call, providing visible warning signs which show the path to preventing serious chronic illness through nutrition. Without my going into explanations, you can easily see the storm at sea here:

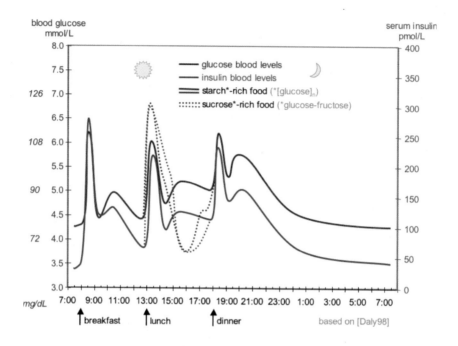

So here again I want to bring us back to the mini-mandala, the epic struggle between cortisol and insulin. Have another look and notice that as the insulin side swells, the cortisol side is stressed and diminishes and as the cortisol side swells, eventually the insulin side can cave, or not. Either way it precedes many chronic illnesses and much unnecessary human suffering. In short, elevated insulin can make us tired while elevated cortisol can diminish insulin function.

On either side, over time, there can be dramatic consequences including chronic fatigue, thyroid dysfunction, immune suppression, hormone imbalance, cardiovascular stress, malabsorption and gut inflammation, headaches including migraines, weight gain, insomnia, depression, kidney stress and liver stress. Additionally, this physiologic storm at sea can lead to aggravation of pre-existing conditions such as fibromyalgia, chronic "subclinical" biofilm infections, autoimmune conditions and cancers.

The Epic Struggle
Insulin/Cortisol

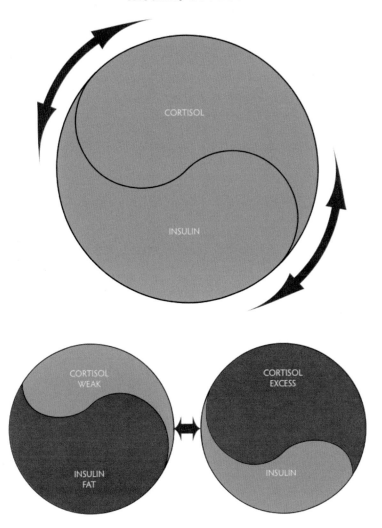

WHAT IS A BIOFILM INFECTION?

Microorganisms that inhabit your body such as bacteria and fungi can live in colonies protected by biofilms. Biofilms serve as a shield to protect the harmful organisms from the immune system and from antibiotic and antifungal medications. Biofilm formation is often the reason why these infections are not easily detectable and medications not always effective.

 ## Take Home Points

- It is important to fill out the glycemic questionnaire in this chapter to determine if imbalanced blood sugar may be causing your symptoms.

- Insulin resistance can happen in anyone due to overconsumption of refined carbohydrates and sugars.

- The increasing demand for more insulin caused by insulin-generating, high-glycemic value foods causes increased abdominal fat accumulation around the waist.

- When necessary, I ask my patients to do a 5-hour glucose tolerance test with serial insulin levels included. I believe it is far more instructive and medically valuable to track serial insulin levels at the same time glucose levels are taken. This test, if indicated, can tell you a lot about your glycemic control, your ability to metabolize sugars and carbohydrates as well as forewarn you about insulin resistance or even borderline diabetes.

- The relationships between glucose levels and insulin levels can provide a person with a valuable wake up call, providing visible warning signs which show the path to preventing serious chronic illness through nutrition.

Your Self-Healing Body in Action

Case Study #3:
Discovering the Root Cause of One Woman's
Chronic Lyme, Endometriosis, Insomnia,
and Other Health Problems

Another case study that illustrates a cloud (mandala) concept of biology and health involves a woman I'll call Diane. We worked together over two years. She has a complicated history that began in late childhood when she was bitten by a tick and contracted what years later was diagnosed as chronic Lyme disease. After the tick bite Diane developed classical symptoms of chronic Lyme, including arthritis as well as a multitude of other symptoms that lasted throughout her teenage years. After two years of a smorgasbord of antibiotics administered both orally and intravenously she seemed to recover from Lyme syndrome, for a time at least.

By the time Diane was fourteen years old she developed endometriosis accompanied by heavy periods with horrendous pain.

Because she had taken many courses of different antibiotics for her Lyme disease, Diane's digestion was compromised (dysbiosis/leaky small bowel/malabsorption). Diane also suffered from polycystic ovary and had all the metabolic imbalances that feed this condition including blood sugar/insulin imbalance, high cortisol demand but diminished capacity to respond (adrenal insufficiency) and gastrointestinal inflammation or IBS (irritable bowel syndrome). All of these conditions could have occurred without Lyme syndrome or multiple antibiotics, but the sum of all the inflammations added to the severity of other conditions even if it was not actually a direct cause. The cloud was a storm cloud. There is no such thing as an isolated event in the body.

When she came to see me, she also noted chronic insomnia accompanied by bruxism (grinding her teeth in her sleep) and subsequent jaw pain and cluster headaches. Furthermore, she had had mononucleosis at age sixteen followed by reoccurring chronic Epstein-Barr virus-related chronic fatigue, mold sensitivities, sinusitis and allergies. All of these problems are holes in the boat that ultimately needed to be addressed to prevent her health from sinking even further into a physiologic storm of inflammation and imbalances.

In spite of all this adversity Diane managed to control her symptoms through her 20s and 30s with a gluten-free, insulin-sparing diet, nutritional therapies including probiotics and a lifestyle that supported her immune system and lowered stress.

When Diane was in her 40s, she had several teeth extracted, dental implants and two root canals within the span of a few months. One of the implants became infected. At the exact same

WHAT IS ENDOMETRIOSIS?

Normally, tissue known as the endometrium lines the inside of a woman's uterus. In endometriosis, this tissue grows outside the uterus instead of inside and yet still acts like tissue growing inside the uterus—it thickens, breaks apart, and bleeds during each menstrual cycle. However, a woman's body can't expel it in the same way as normal tissue lining the inside of the uterus. Consequently, it becomes trapped. When there is ovarian involvement, scarring can occur and fibrous tissue can form, causing pelvic tissue and organs to adhere to each other. Often, this is an extremely painful condition.

time, her Lyme disease reactivated, more than twenty-five years after her tick bite. She started feeling symptoms she had not experienced in years. Her endometriosis also worsened and her abdomen became bloated and painful. Her menstrual cycles were heavy and incapacitating, filled with abdominal spams that started a week or more before and continued through her menstrual period. Her gynecologist eventually ordered a CA-125 test, a marker for ovarian cancer. Although the test was strongly positive, no scan or specialist could find any sign of a tumor. All of these issues began within several months of her dental work and dental infection. The dam had burst and her body was decompensating.

> ## ABOUT THE CA-125 TEST
>
> *A CA-125 test is used to detect the protein CA 125 (cancer antigen 125). It is used to measure progress during and after treatment of certain cancers and to detect early signs of ovarian cancer, especially in women at high risk of the disease. CA 125 can become elevated for a number of reasons including menstruation and noncancerous conditions such as uterine fibroids. Therefore, it is not a stand-alone way to screen for ovarian cancer.*

A Destructive Pattern

When taking on complex cases like Diane's, where there is not only inflammation but also debilitation, the road signs all say, *"Go Slow, Dangerous Curves."* We need to listen carefully to a person's story and proceed slowly and carefully. I believe the best way to approach chronic illness is close observation, striving whenever possible to use the sophistication of the body's own healing capacity to promote a healing pattern. Sometimes successful healing is difficult to accomplish due to inherited traits that allow inflammation to dominate. Other times there are blocking conditions in the form of toxicities, infections and other imbalances or deficiencies that don't allow healing to proceed. The body is stuck in a ditch, spinning its wheels. An individual's biology is something that can be best appreciated by listening carefully—family history, personal history from pre-birth to present. By listening carefully over an hour or two we can pick up nuances that give clues not only about what is happening, but also how it happens and maybe why it happens.

After a long session and sometimes two sessions one can form a good understanding of what needs to be addressed, how to prioritize various layers of issues as well as which therapies a person might best respond to. I always look at the hypoglycemic questionnaire that my patients fill out. Patients rate items on the questionnaire from 0 to 3 in terms of the severity on a list of over thirty symptoms such as craving sugar, feeling tired after meals, getting shaky and hungry, irritability, emotional volatility, clarity of thought and sleep patterns. After reviewing this list I'll ask a series of questions: "What time do you go to bed, what time do you get up? What do you eat? What's the first thing you do when you get up in the morning?" And then I'll ask about a patient's energy levels at those times. "How's your energy at noon? How's your energy after you eat? When do you experience a crash time in the afternoon? How do you sleep?" An overall picture emerges from the responses to this line of questioning that paints a more complete picture of circadian rhythms and vitality.

Diane's pattern was fatigue in the morning. She would drink some coffee and maybe a fruit smoothie. Then she would have a minimal lunch and crash in the afternoon. She acted this way because she always felt worse after eating, so to avoid one set of problems she caused others. In the evening, her energy returned. She'd fall asleep at night but then she awakened at 3 a.m. and couldn't fall back to sleep. That's a corrosive pattern in and of itself and it was fed by the fact that she was eating quite a bit of refined carbs due to hypoglycemia caused cravings. High-glycemic foods with high sugar content such as refined grains, sugars, fruit juices and candy act like jet fuel—in other words, they're fast burning and they're pro-inflammatory. She was growing more and more depleted. There were many old holes in the boat, but also a physiologic storm at sea brewing. Diane's body was unable to find a firm base to rebuild. She was just trying to keep her head above water, bailing out symptoms with diminishing success and energy.

The first step we took was to reduce her stress load by stabilizing blood sugar and encouraging better absorption. I recommended that she return to eating non-inflammatory, lower glycemic foods. She was to eat smaller meals more frequently including more protein. We also started Diane on a few supplements such as chromium picolinate, alpha-lipoic acid and some digestive enzymes with betaine hydrochloride to improve digestion and correct hypoglycemic patterns. She also started taking water with l-glutamine powder and a little vitamin C. The amino acid l-glutamine is critical for repairing leaky gut as well as reducing sugar cravings, crashes and muscle wasting. Vitamin C supports the adrenals. Together with probiotics these nutrients were Diane's rescue remedy. Resolving blood sugar imbalance and afternoon cortisol-linked energy crashes act to calm symptoms including brain fog and agitation, reduce cortisol demand and create a level playing field for the body to turn chaos into rebuilding and healing. Once these stormy layers have started to resolve over a week or two, many symptoms fade or go away completely. New symptoms sometimes emerge while some old symptoms remain. Symptoms that remain point the way towards the next stage of therapy needed. It is here we can begin to judge where anatomical and physiologic blockages exist. After many of the physiologic storm symptoms subside, the deeper, more primary issues are exposed and can be more effectively addressed. We can begin to address repairing some of the holes in the boat. Diane could begin to heal at deeper levels.

After resolving glycemic issues, Diane's energy level began to improve, her thinking was more clear and focused, she definitely felt less overwhelmed by daily challenges, she could see the negative feedback loops she had become entangled in. Nothing had changed in a profound way, yet, Diane just felt better and gained confidence that her body could

SLOW-BURNING, LOW-GLYCEMIC FOODS

The foods you eat are given a glycemic index score. The higher the glycemic index, the more the food raises blood sugar levels. However, the glycemic index is not considered the most accurate way to measure a food's effect on blood sugar. Glycemic load is a more accurate measurement because it paints a more complete picture of a food's effect on blood sugar. The glycemic load measures the rate at which the food causes a spike in blood sugar and the amount of glucose that food will deliver. A food with a score of 10 or below has a low-glycemic load whereas foods with a score of 20 or higher are best avoided. You can find a table of the glycemic index and glycemic load of common foods at http://www.health. harvard.edu/diseases-and-conditions/glycemic_index_and_glycemic_load_for_100_foods heal. At first, resisting refined carbs is an uphill challenge, but after a brief time, cravings for sugar diminish. Eating lower glycemic foods is like putting kindling and hardwood on the fire rather than using paper; energy cycles stabilize, cortisol demand diminishes, sleep patterns improve and a feeling of calm settles in.

Resolving hypoglycemia allows our brains to think clearly and calmly. The brain cannot store glucose so it's dependent on our fuel intake, absorption and the stored energy in the liver, muscles and other organs. The way the brain signals low blood sugar states is by telling the body, "burn the furniture, there's no fuel." In other words, there is a shock response and this shock response involves cortisol. Cortisol tells the liver and the muscles, joints and tendons to give up stored energy because the brain and nervous system are in trouble. The body prioritizes its metabolism according to what's in front of it. If it's on survival mode it will do things that prioritize quick release of energy at the expense of other organs and structures. With her blood sugar more stable, Diane also experienced less bloating and gas and better absorption of and response to some nutrients. Probiotics, anti-inflammatory aloe vera and glutamine all combined to help. The sympathetic (flight/fight) aspect of Diane's autonomic nervous system was less stressed so her parasympathetic internal organ functions including digestive capacity began to improve as well. The knots began to unravel.

A Roadblock to Success

Addressing Diane's glycemic problems allowed her to repair. It allowed her to feel better, which is important. Improving blood sugar was the easiest way to remove some of Diane's stress. If you stabilize blood sugar you put the brain on an even playing field and suddenly, your digestion is better, sleep is better and energy starts coming back. With just a little flip, that turns a downward, worsening spiral into an upward, healing spiral. She gained some confidence that she could heal.

Many underlying reasons behind the holes in the boat still needed to be addressed, however. When Diane first came to my office I examined her dental X-rays and noticed dental implants and root canals. I suggested she visit a dentist specializing in assessing dental root, gum and bone health (an endodontist) in order to have a CBCT, a CT scan of the upper and lower jaw and teeth. The CBCT provides a three-dimensional image of the facial bones, the upper and lower palettes, the teeth and their roots. Using this type of imaging device, silent infections under root canals can be detected more accurately. Root canaled teeth are essentially dead teeth. Root canaled teeth lack dental pulp or nerve innervation so there is usually no pain associated with silent degenerative infections deep in and around roots. When accurately read, the CBCT can illuminate areas of focal infection, immune challenge and stress on the body's healing capacity. Diane resisted doing this scan at first. The thought of revisiting dental issues is often very daunting.

We continued Diane's nutritional/digestive support but she continued to limp along, at times much better, at times feeling worse. Often the worst times coincided with her menstrual cycles. A trail of medical problems continued to follow her. However, none of the treatments Diane used resulted in any long-term success. Finally, I convinced Diane to have the dental scan. And once she did things began to change for the better and more permanently.

The Root Cause of Her Problems

I took one look at the dental scan and the analysis and told Diane, "I can understand now why all your various issues have not been able to resolve more permanently." The CBCT report diagnosed several chronic, bone-eroding infections in her jaw. They were a constant immune challenge that diminished Diane's infection-fighting capacity to bacteria and to viruses. These infections were eroding her vitality and blocking her body's ability to heal itself in spite of all the positive things she was doing. Her body's immune system was like a car battery getting worn down after the car alarm had been on for 12 hours.

From the dental scan, it was obvious that one of the implants had penetrated up into the maxillary sinus and likely behind her chronic sinus infections. The scan also revealed she had an infected root canal. Luckily, three of the upper implants were not infected. But there were signs of an infection on an implant on the lower teeth. The erosion of bone at the root of and a dead tooth was silently poisoning Diane's immune system with cadaverous bacteria and leaking those bacteria and bacterial endotoxins into her bloodstream. We decided it was time to act to eliminate these challenges.

A Dramatic Improvement

Diane went to an expert dental surgeon to correct these dental issues, including extraction of the root-canaled molar that had gone bad. We used craniosacral release techniques to help release the tension and clenching of her jaw muscles. Resolving her dental infection and stabilizing her blood sugar both helped reduce her stress/cortisol loads. Diane's clenching improved, her headaches diminished, her body pains including her menstrual cycle PMS and cramping diminished, thyroid antibodies and hypothyroid symptoms abated and finally, her digestion and blood sugar instability improved even more than before.

After addressing the dental issues, Diane began a series of detoxification/elimination and immune-strengthening therapies. Her improvements were dramatic. Her sinusitis and allergies improved and her sinuses were

> ## ABOUT CRANIOSACRAL THERAPY
>
> *In craniosacral therapy, the skull is gently manipulated in order to reduce pain and tension. The technique supports central nervous system function.*

much less reactive. Her periods became substantially less painful. Prior to the dental work and other therapies Diane was taking 12-hour Advil® twice daily for a week before and then during her menstrual cycles. After the dental work and subsequent therapies, she required only one Advil® the first day of her period. Her bloating went down and her digestion improved partly because less anti-inflammatory over-the-counter pain meds (NSAIDs or nonsteroidal anti-inflammatory drugs) allowed gut inflammation to heal. In addition, her joint pain was nearly gone.

An interesting aside here is that the teeth that had been involved with Diane's implants and root canals were related energetically to the pancreas, the ovaries and kidney stone formation on what is called an Odonton dental chart. This is a system that originated in German and Oriental naturopathic medical traditions and that relates acupuncture channels with organ function. The Odonton maps out tooth/channel/organ connections. Similar holographic mapping occurs in acupuncture tradition on the ears, tongue, nose, feet and hands. In Western medicine there are a few such correlations recorded including shoulder blade pain with a gallstone attack. Few things in biology have one-to-one correlations with absolute precision or consistency but the holography of our bodies never ceases to amaze me. When we look and listen carefully we will learn.

> **WHAT IS AN ODONTON?**
>
> *Odonton refers to the connection that exists between the teeth and other areas of your body. Problems that occur in certain teeth are associated with the development of disease in a corresponding area of the body.*

When I encounter really complicated cases, when the patient is doing all the right things and still not getting enough response, I look for deep-seated focal blockages. Focal blockages do not allow our body to resolve inflammations or disease processes. They are big boulders in the road that obstruct our self-healing potential. In addressing focal blockages our body can begin to resolve that impasse. By eliminating impasses, the body can move to another level of immune function, of vitality and of healing. Having all those dental implants done at the same time was a real shock to Diane's system that reactivated pre-existing conditions. Diane's case is an excellent warning to us all: *don't overlook dental health.* Diane's healing voyage continues; she still suffers from lesser symptoms of endometriosis and may require more medical intervention, as well as ongoing health maintenance, but her course to improved quality of life, to following her passions and professional interests and reclaiming her life is well underway.

Making Medicine More Personal

Physicians have too often given over what they know best about patient care to insurance companies and HMO dictates. It's past time for physicians to have the courage to take the practice of medicine back. It's past time physicians offer their patients better standards and more time for listening for those interested. In the late 1950s it was argued that third party insurance payments were "immoral," that physicians owed their patients person-to-person consideration, attention and care. It is a personal relationship that matters most. The "7-minute consultation" is anathema to the best practice of good patient care and relationship. Both the patient and the physician are left dissatisfied and unheard. Disease focus and treatments, surgical innovations and the biological sciences have and continue to carve out necessary and distinguished places in the history of medicine. Beyond this, pathologically oriented medicine has poor models for addressing and interpreting the multiple stress vectors resulting in most chronic degenerative illnesses. Its focus has been on pathology vs. dysfunctional physiology. There is an artificial divide of body and mind, physiology and emotions. In fact, these divisions are human word constructs intended to wrap our brains around the complexity of Nature.

When you dissolve these dichotomies, when you dissolve these artificial categories which restrict your problem-solving capacity and tie you to past failures, you open yourself and your children to understanding your true self-healing capacity. You can begin to appreciate neurotransmitters, holographic feedback and the interconnectedness of all your body's organs, structures and systems and the debilitating corrosiveness of cortisol overload over time.

Not taking on the intellectual task of understanding and applying interactive, holographic system models to the practice of medicine is a major failing of contemporary medical education. Quantum physics is used every day in CT scans, MRIs and other advanced yet commonly used medical technologies, and yet, often medical thinking is grounded in mechanistic 19th Century physics and linear, cause-effect paradigms. These failings cannot be compensated for by weekend seminars filled with Cartesian pigeonholed *fix-its* using vitamin/herbal formulas any more than pharmaceuticals. If your diagnostic paradigms cannot embrace complexity and emergence then you will never begin to appreciate complex biological systems, you will get on the wrong train and never arrive at the right destination no matter how fast and flashy a train you're on. In the meantime, when you're out walking, look up at the clouds and sky, think about your place in the quantum levels above and below that make us happen and connect with the beauty of your self-healing body.

ADDENDUM

About the Current Direction of Medicine

Medicine has become a library of diagnostic codes in search of insurance payments, and people serving medicine rather than medicine serving people.

Telemedicine has become the new norm—convenient, hygienic and less messy than face-to-face encounters. This new norm has blossomed during a pandemic but also fits corporate financial models of efficiency, as well as the desire for speed and quick fixes—in short, superficial but more profitable.

Try getting an oil and filter change on a Zoom meeting. Medicine, at its highest level, is both science and an art. To maximize benefits, it requires all the senses, especially hands on attention to careful physical examination. It also takes time to reveal and fathom signs and symptoms along with the story of the person behind them. How often do physicians look at test results then glance at their patient to imply or say outright, "but everything looks normal, you look fine on paper." I would say this is a common interaction, conveying disbelief and causing their patient to feel discarded on a scrap pile of missed opportunity for healing. We are decades overdue for physicians to take back the practice of medicine.

Please Review This Book on Amazon

I want to help your friends and family remove their blocks to optimal health. Please help spread the word about this book by reviewing it on Amazon and posting the Amazon book link on your social media pages. We're all interconnected, and it is only with your help that this important information will fall into the hands of the people who need it the most.

About the Author

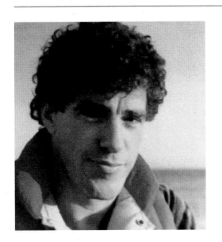

DANIEL DUNPHY has been a practicing clinician in nutritionally oriented family medical practice since 1980. His most important teachers have been his many patients to whom he owes endless thanks. For more information and to access the free interactive Holosystemic Mandala App, visit **www.biomedarts.com**

Made in the USA
Columbia, SC
22 July 2023

20720945R00073